HOW TO SURVIVE YOUR DOCTOR'S CARE

PAMELA F. GALLIN, M.D., F.A.C.S.

HOW TO SURVIVE YOUR DOCTOR'S CARE

Get the Right Diagnosis, the Right
Treatment, and the Right Experts for You

PAMELA F. GALLIN, M.D., F.A.C.S.

LifeLine
Press®

A Regnery Publishing Company, Washington, D.C.

Library of Congress Cataloging-in-Publication Data on file.

ISBN 0-89526-120-0

Published in the United States by
LifeLine Press
A Regnery Publishing Company
One Massachusetts Avenue, N.W.
Washington, DC 20001

Visit us at www.lifelinepress.com

Distributed to the trade by
National Book Network
4720-A Boston Way
Lanham, MD 20706

Printed on acid-free paper
Manufactured in the United States of America

10 9 8 7 6 5 4 3 2

Books are available in quantity for promotional or premium use. Write to Director of Special Sales, Regnery Publishing, Inc., One Massachusetts Avenue, N.W., Washington, DC 20001, for information on discounts and terms or call (202) 216-0600.

The information contained in this book is not a substitute for medical counseling and care. All matters pertaining to your physical health should be supervised by a health care professional.

In honor of my teachers,
Ronnie and Sharon Burde,
who by example taught me to be
a wife, mother, and physician.

CONTENTS

Foreword   **ix**
Acknowledgments   **xi**
Introduction   **xiii**

Foreword

MEDICAL CARE AT ITS BEST in the United States is the best in the world. Yet despite this fact, or even because of it, patients can be confused and overwhelmed when it comes to visiting the doctor. Along with the best technology and trained specialists, patients are faced with a dizzying array of medical opinions and treatment options—not to mention the complex web of managed care.

As a result, today's patients need to be more informed and involved than ever before. In her lively and informative way, Dr. Pamela Gallin writes that in order to receive the best care—to survive *and thrive* in medical care—every one of us must become active participants in our own care. Through helpful advice and telling anecdotes, Dr. Gallin outlines the ways to educate and empower ourselves through every aspect of care, from diagnosis to second opinions to medical emergencies.

The single most important decision for a patient, says Dr. Gallin, is choosing the right hospital or medical center. Your doctor is one part of a larger organization with specialists, technicians, nurses, and other care providers, each of whom can be vital to your good health. Choosing the right "home" for your care also means choosing a place that treats you as a person, helps you feel comfortable, and allows you to best understand and make use of the resources it offers.

I am confident that this book will help countless patients and their families form informed partnerships with their doctors, fostering superior communication and superior care.

HERBERT PARDES, M.D.
President and CEO
New York-Presbyterian Hospital
New York, New York

Acknowledgments

THIS BOOK IS THE CONTINUATION of an education I began at Washington University in St. Louis, where I was transformed by my professors into a physician. Dr. Ronald Burde, Dr. Morton Smith, and the entire faculty of the Washington University School of Medicine participated in my education directly through their invaluable scientific knowledge and by showing me how to become a caring physician.

Later, when I was an intern at New York University Medical Center and then a Mt. Sinai Medical Center resident, Drs. Steven Podos, Maurice Luntz, Robert Ritch, Murray Meltzer, and other faculty invested their time and energy into my education. Drs. Philip Knapp and Marshall Parks, who are both renowned in my field for their intelligence, expertise, compassion, surgical skills, and judgment, sculpted my subspecialty. Without them I would not exist: They are my heredity.

It makes me proud to be a member of the faculty of Columbia-Presbyterian Medical Center (New York-Presbyterian), led by Herbert Pardes, M.D., an able leader and visionary.

We work as a team. The physician ideal is based on a composite of doctors: Amy Newburger, Howard Newburger, John

Driscoll, Yvonne Driscoll, Harry Lodge, John Postley, Laura Corio, Allen Hyman, Mark Sultan, Joseph Levy, Charles Stolar, Peter Altman, David Roye, Lynn Quitell, Myles Behrens, Michael Kazim, Arthur Cotliar, George Florakis, Hermann Schubert, Marc Odrich, Steve Trokel, and many others with whom I have had the privilege to interact. And to Cynthia Sparer, who makes it all run.

Brian Dotson at all times has been my champion, advisor, and advocate. His gentle prodding has been invaluable. Myrna Manners smoothed the path with the support of New York-Presbyterian, which she epitomizes.

Many of the faculty reviewed chapters and made important modifications: Arlene Trykko, R.N.; Charles Marboe, M.D.; Lena Sun, M.D.; Robert Kazim, M.D.; Myles Behrens, M.D.; Jeffrey Odel, M.D.; and Ralph Green, M.D., were quite helpful.

Judy Schwartz put ideas and concepts into words and phrases, always with kindness and judgment. To Judy, I am grateful.

Daily, Mary Michaels graciously and seamlessly organized the pieces of this large puzzle.

LifeLine Press is a unique organization. Mike Ward's foresight, Marji Ross's supervision, and Molly Mullen's direct vision brought this to fruition, at times amidst adversity. Lauren Lawson has made the book known to all—and cheered me on. Beth Mottar put all the pieces in order and made it cohesive. With humor, John Lalor helped negotiate the distribution of this book and has been an enthusiastic supporter.

And my magnificent family, Leonard, Laura, Abigail, Hilary, and Peter, who make life joyous—and are my daily instructors. They initiated, cajoled, cheered, modified, and were the template for this effort.

Most of all, I am appreciative to the many personal friends, family members, and patients who allowed their stories to be told, all in an attempt to help the reader benefit from the best medical care in the world—that in the USA.

Introduction

MY STORY

About six years into my surgical career, I developed a joint inflammation in my right hand. As I am a right-handed surgeon, this was not a good thing. The build-up of inflammatory debris fused two of the little bones together, and I couldn't bend my hand. I could manage small hand movements, like picking up a pencil and, at least for the time being, I was able to operate, but large hand movements were out. I couldn't, for instance, unscrew a peanut butter jar—rather an inconvenience as I had four children under ten.

I did all the things a good patient should do. I got opinions from three surgeons who specialized in hand surgery. All offered the same verdict: I needed an operation to alleviate the inflammation. I chose the surgeon who had the most experience in hand surgery. He was a respected academic physician who himself trained world-famous surgeons. I couldn't have asked for more.

Or so I thought.

The surgery itself went smoothly. After a night in the hospital, the surgeon pronounced me fine and sent me home with my hand in a cast and an appointment to be seen in six weeks.

When I got home my hand started to hurt—a lot. Nobody had given me an indication of how much pain to expect, so I wasn't sure whether this was typical. But I have a fairly high threshold for pain and this was truly unbearable. I ordered a narcotic to ease the pain, which, in retrospect, was the wrong thing to do: The pain was my body's way of telling me that something wasn't right, and the medication merely masked the problem.

I called the surgeon and told him I was in a lot of pain. He assured me that I was fine and no doubt overreacting. I thought: What was I, a wimp? I felt like a student who had disappointed her teacher.

Despite his promises, the pain did not go away. In fact, it got worse.

The cast went just to the top of my fingers, and after three days of calling the surgeon to no avail, my fingers swelled up like little sausages. I spoke to a radiologist friend, who urged me to demand an appointment. That Friday I did what I should have done the first day: I called and told the surgeon's secretary that I wanted to be seen. She replied flatly that he was out of town. (As it turned out, he was attending a party honoring him for being such a fine surgeon and teacher.) I told her I didn't care, I'd see someone else.

I went to another surgeon, also a professor. He looked at my hand and literally ripped the cast off. Though he didn't say anything, I could tell he was furious. At that moment, I realized I wasn't being unreasonable. There really *was* something wrong. The cast had been put on too tightly so that the top of it pressed down across the base of my hand, impeding the blood supply and squashing the nerves.

Once the crisis settled down, I got angry. The surgeon's lack of response had made me feel there was something wrong with me, that I was a bad patient. In retrospect, he made me feel as if I was seen as an hysterical woman. The fact that I was a surgical colleague—and a right-handed one at that—made his indifference that much more enraging and insulting. But he should have tended to me no matter who I was. If he was too busy, another surgeon could have seen me.

When, weeks later, I went back to the surgeon who had put the cast on, his manner had changed completely. He couldn't have been more solicitous. By his attitude, I knew that my post-operative hand problem was worse than I thought. Ultimately, I went to a neurologist, who confirmed that I had nerve damage in the skin of my hand. It took six months for the nerves to grow back.

Understand, the operation itself had been a success. But because the surgeon didn't listen to me about the pain, a too-tight cast remained on for five days and the incision popped open. Due to the swelling under the cast, I also wound up with a very thick scar, called a keloid. It was unbecoming, to say the least. But worst of all, every day it reminded me of what had happened. Over the next two years I underwent two scar revisions by a fine plastic surgeon who specializes in hands. Each time I was in a cast for a month.

In the end, the problem was fixed. But much of what I went through—days of excruciating pain, persisting nerve damage, the inconvenience and expense of subsequent surgery—would not have happened had the surgeon listened to me and treated me with respect.

Nor would this have happened had I had the strength of conviction to challenge the surgeon the day after the surgery. The lesson I learned—and what I hope you will take from this story—is that if a little voice goes off in your head saying that something is wrong, have the doctor see you. Don't take no for an answer. Granted, it's a natural response to back down when someone in authority questions you. But don't let yourself be cowed, as I was initially.

Even after two rounds of plastic surgery, I still have a small scar, a little white line that runs across the top of my hand. Most people don't even notice it. But I do.

It's a permanent reminder to speak up when I feel something is not right.

POWER TO THE PATIENT

You may be wondering why I am telling you this. To tell you that doctors make mistakes? In part, but you probably already knew that. I share this story to help you find the safe, quality care you need. After all, if someone with all my medical connections and expertise can get caught up short, I thought, what about the ordinary person for whom hospitals, surgery, and diagnosis are alien turf?

Many people dear to me, in my personal and professional life, do not know how to find the right doctor for what troubles them. These are competent, intelligent people who are quite savvy in most areas of their lives. But to many people, perhaps most, the maze that today's medical system represents is confusing and overwhelming. In a sense, every profession is a conspiracy against the layman. But as the guardian of our physical well-being, the medical profession affects each of us profoundly.

I have learned a great deal as a medical student, wife, mother, patient, and surgeon at one of the nation's leading medical centers. I have found that there is a logic to the medical care system—a logic that may not be immediately apparent to someone outside of it. In this book, I want to share what I know so that you will have a framework within which to understand any medical scenarios that you confront. Many of you are out there trying your best to get good care for yourselves and for family members and feel outright stumped by the system. With a little bit of information, with perhaps someone privy to the ways of medicine whispering in your ear, you can learn the route to consistently good care. I want to tell you what the system is like, as seen from the inside. Let me be that person whispering in your ear. I would like this knowledge to inspire and to empower you to seek and secure the best medical care available—the care that you deserve.

Now more than ever, the onus is on the patient to ensure that he receives proper medical treatment. In the past, people generally had the same doctor over many years, and they trusted his advice. If this doctor said, "Do this," they would do it without a qualm. Today, the directives may come from a managed care company or from a doctor you've just signed on with because the insurance provider list has changed and your previous doctor is not on it. However, the factors we all commonly complain about, such as hospital bureaucracies, cost containment, increased specialization, and HMOs, are only partly responsible for the current, complicated state of medical care. Medicine itself is now more sophisticated, with new knowledge, technology, and treatment possibilities being introduced by the day.

In medicine today, everything is sped up. The volume of diagnostic tests, procedures, and patient visits has increased. If there is, say, one error in a lab test, that error will be compounded as the patient moves through the course of treatment. As patients, we need to be more vigilant. The fact is that the faster we go and the more pieces of information involved, the greater chance that we'll be struck by friendly fire—that a diagnosis or test intended to help a patient will instead deliver further harm.

It's tempting to blame the doctors for less than perfect medicine, but modern medical care has doctors themselves up in arms. Due to a confluence of forces beyond an individual doctor's control, physicians have little choice but to do more, go faster, and spread themselves thinner. That does not, however, mean that mistakes are okay.

Nor do you always need to accept the care that's being offered to you. With cost containment on everybody's mind, medical professionals are sometimes pushed beyond the limits of their training and expertise. You need to understand what you're getting, feel that you can challenge the care presented, and know that you can make demands.

Recently, my daughter, away at college, injured both of her ankles and went to the emergency room of her university, which happened to be a medical school. She was seen by a nurse practitioner, who said that it was a sprain. According to the X-ray, there was no bone damage. But she was in excruciating pain. The next day she saw an orthopedist, a specialist who could observe the subtleties of the problem. He confirmed her feelings that the injury was more severe than the nurse practitioner had indicated: She had two torn ligaments in one ankle, one in the other, and bone spurs in both heels. My daughter had been given crutches but not a brace, which she needed. The nurse practitioner should have seen that this case went beyond her territory and called in an orthopedist. She should have passed the baton. But due to time, financial, and personnel constraints, she was under pressure to run with it. Had my daughter understood this, she could have demanded to see an orthopedist or, at the very least, the emergency room physician.

Medicine is a consumer issue. We physicians are service providers. We work for *you*—not the other way around. Over the last ten to fifteen years, the issue of patient rights has come to the fore. Patients are more aware that their medical records belong to them and have a better understanding of what it means to sign a consent form. Evincing this progress, the *Patient Bill of Rights*—a document worth acquainting yourself with (see page 218)—is posted prominently in every hospital in the country.

Good medical care is a right, not a privilege. Know that. Many think that they can't get good care because they're not entitled to it. The truth is many people would walk out of a store if they received the same treatment they may have received in a doctor's office. They think that if they were a CEO or a celebrity, they'd be entitled to expect good treatment. The system seems to be stacked against the individual, with entry only to those in the know. But wealth, status, or connections do not guarantee fine care. It's how you set up your own health care that determines its quality. And this book can help you do it correctly.

Your doctors want to help you. Know that, too. Men and women go into medicine because they want to alleviate suffering and are willing to dedicate their lives to that aim. When I speak to medical students, I say, "Look, doctors are getting hammered these days. Are you sorry that you're doing this?" Their response is, "No, this is what we want to do." Many have tried the business world or other professions and decided that only working to heal others would give their lives meaning. I hear this again and again. It makes me optimistic about medicine. The occasional cavalier attitude or the odd rogue that may be out there are exceptions rather than the rule. And this book will tell you how to avoid those.

I believe deeply in the virtues of American medicine. In this country, we are blessed with the best medical care in the world, and I have seen the best that medicine can do; that is the standard to which I adhere. I know that level of excellence is out there— and that you can have it. When everything comes together and, through surgery, medication, and astute diagnosis, someone is brought back to glowing health, it is nothing short of miraculous. However, my own uncomfortable loss of innocence has forced me to confront the fact that all doesn't always go right. I would like to be honest about the medical field's shortcomings so that others can avoid potentially dangerous situations. The idealism I still have about medicine, along with my belief in a patient's right to information, has led me to share what I know, to spell out how to get the fine care that I know is out there.

How to Survive Your Doctor's Care is intended as a primer on how to decode the medical system, from an insider's vantage point. I'll explain how things work, why they work that way, and what that means to you, the medical consumer. I'll tell you how to get to the doctors you deserve and the care that you need.

This book speaks to people in good health, for the best time to organize your medical care is when you're healthy. When you're ill, everything becomes more urgent, so you may have less leeway and fewer options; also, you may not think very clearly when you're not feeling well. If you plan ahead, however, everything is in place for the occasion when you *do* get sick.

And certainly, this book will be useful to people in the throes of medical decision-making—when you or a family member is seeking or has received a diagnosis or when you're deciding between treatments or considering surgery. While it's best to be plugged into the system before a medical crisis, this book will help you deal strategically with what you're confronting.

PART ONE

FUNDAMENTALS

CHAPTER ONE

A Doctor's-Eye View of Medicine

T
HERE IS A UNIQUE "DOCTOR'S WAY" of looking at the health care system. This singular perspective is formed by their training, their understanding of the hierarchy, and what they've absorbed from living amidst the medical culture. You can learn about this culture much the way that an anthropologist studies a remote, unexplored society. Indeed, it is like a separate society, with its own universally acknowledged codes, milestones, and rites of passage. As someone on the receiving end of medical care, learning to view medicine through the doctor's lens will give you an inside peek into the medical system. It will also help you work with your doctor, for you will better understand his or her decision-making process, goals, and constraints.

There are four main features that distinguish the medical culture. These are (1) the importance of apprenticeship features; (2) the hierarchy within the field; (3) the code of respect among physicians; and (4) the certification system. Although these attributes are invisible to the general public, each has an effect on the medical care that you receive.

APPRENTICESHIP

Contrary to the stereotype of doctors as aloof, scientific sorts, usually too busy for chit-chat, medicine is, as much as anything, a profession based on personal relationships. I'm not saying that doctors per se are gregarious or like to schmooze, but that a physician's career is built over time from significant mentoring and working relationships. One moves from being a student who's never even held a scalpel to a competent, assured physician through apprenticeships to more accomplished physicians. Knowledgeable generalists and specialists take fledgling doctors under wing, devoting a great deal of time and energy to the young doctors' development. In doing so, experienced doctors put their stamp on the next generation of doctors, passing along their knowledge, technique, and standards.

It's really quite an old-fashioned system. Years ago, the route into any trade or profession—everything from silversmithing to masonry to banking—was a long apprenticeship. Medicine's apprenticeship model isn't anything secretive, but it occurs beyond public view. I'm here to offer you a glimpse into the depth and importance of these relationships by demonstrating how they were important to me.

THE BIRTH OF A DOCTOR

First of all, I didn't decide to become a doctor; my professors at Washington University in St. Louis decided that for me. I wasn't one of those small children who walked around with a toy stethoscope around my neck. My plan was to graduate from college, get a job in engineering (my area of study), and perhaps get married. But at Washington University, there was a close connection between the medical school and the undergraduate programs. The idea was to give students an opportunity to see what other fields and majors were like. This was in the early 1970s, when computerization was just starting to be applied to medicine. Washington University had one of the nation's first computerized surgical intensive care units, set up by the engineering school's biomedical computer lab. The overlap between engineering and medicine made perfect sense. I didn't realize it at the time, but in taking that route, I took my first step toward a medical career. By observing and emulating the people above me, I was learning to think as a doctor.

As a sophomore, I took a minicourse called "Hearts and Parts: The Engineering of Artificial Organs," one of those classes offered to give students a taste of what medicine was all about. As part of the course, I performed corneal transplants on rabbits. The first time, it took me thirty minutes to put one suture through the poor rabbit's eye. To put this in perspective, a corneal transplant is typically completed in about forty-five minutes, with about thirty sutures in all. The resident assigned to guide me through this formidable task is now among the world's leading cornea experts. I still see him on occasion at professional gatherings. We both laugh about that first surgery—and about the fact that I wound up as an ophthalmologist in spite of it.

As inauspicious as my debut may have been, it was the beginning for me. The cornea project, it turned out, was related to work the young resident was doing for Ronald Burde, M.D., an extraordinary man who eventually went on to hold an unheard-of four full professorships: in Ophthalmology, Neurosurgery, Neurology, and Medicine. Through the resident's instruction, and later through his own work with me, I was the beneficiary of Dr. Burde's hard-earned knowledge. That experience taught me one of the cardinal rules of the apprenticeship model: When you have expertise, you teach it to the person coming along behind you. It's your obligation to do so. Every experienced physician has a responsibility to those in training; it's part of the unwritten code.

I soon discovered mentors among other residents at the medical center. I reveled in their company. I found myself swept up in the excitement of medicine—the thrill of learning highly complex material and then applying it to an actual person and making them better. It was at once intellectual, action-oriented, and altru-istic. In me, the residents saw potential and an excitement that mirrored their own. They spent precious time with me sharing what they knew—the subtle language of rank, the secrets of the trade. As they let me tag along with them at lunch, I found myself privy to discussions of complex medical cases and dilemmas.

I remember one occasion when that first ophthalmology resi-dent was anxious about a case. While operating on a three-year-old child, he had found what he thought was a life-threatening tumor. Using his best clinical judgment, he decided to remove the eye. He was now awaiting the ophthalmic pathologist's report. He would soon learn that he had either saved this child's life or unnecessarily removed an eye. With great concern, he told Dr. Morton Smith, a respected colleague, about the case. Dr. Smith reassured him that, based on the information available at the time, he had made the right decision. Still, the possibility that he had made the wrong decision weighed heavily on him. I watched the drama unfold; the report confirmed that his judgment had been correct. It made quite an impression that this resident doc-tor, whom I respected greatly, had revealed such deeply held doubt and apprehension in my presence.

Officially, I was still in the Engineering School, but residents and professors started saying to me, "Why don't you go to med-ical school?" adding that they thought I'd make a good doctor. My reaction was, "Huh, me?" Until then, it had never occurred to me. To assume I could actually be a doctor seemed presump-tuous. But I was eventually won over. After seeing how doctors worked at a major medical center, I decided I wanted to try to be like those doctors if they would have me as a student. At first, I considered getting a Ph.D. in biomedical computer engineering, but I soon realized that would keep me on the periphery of the world I found so exciting.

I can still remember exactly when the decision to become a doctor crystallized for me. I was standing in line at the dormitory lunchroom. The girl ahead of me was someone I knew casually, certainly not well enough for me to put my fate in her hands. Yet, out of the blue, I said to her, "Do you think I'd be a decent doctor?"

"Yes," she said. "I think you'd be a very fine doctor."

"Really?"

That spurred me on. If she had said no, I likely would have shelved the whole idea. Thus life-changing decisions are made.

APPRENTICESHIP IN ACTION

I entered medical school as one of two dozen female members of my class. Washington University was so proud that its entering class was one-quarter women that it put a photo of us on the cover of the medical school alumni magazine. Now that at least half of all medical students are women, this doesn't seem so remarkable. But at the time, the mid-1970s, this was very progressive; there were only six the year before, and fewer each year before that. We felt special and empowered. It's worth noting, however, that competition for the few slots earmarked for women was exceedingly rigorous. So opening the doors to women didn't necessarily translate into greater opportunities for most women, or, for that matter, for minorities.

Once I was inside the system, my professors wanted me to succeed. They wanted this for me, not for me "as a woman." Succeeding didn't mean just getting good grades. They wanted me to be like them, to do what they did, and to emulate them. They wanted me to carry on their work and their approach. It is a privilege when somebody says, "I'm going to train you." There were a number of physicians who invested their time and effort in me. That personal attention continued from my four years in college through four years in medical school and another five years as an intern, resident, and fellow.

I can describe my medical lineage quite specifically; it is an integral part of who I am as a physician. It starts with Dr. Burde,

a truly gifted teacher and physician. His teaching and sage coun-
sel helped me, in my third year of medical school, choose ophthalmology over neurosurgery as my specialty, a decision I've
never regretted. I enjoy doing fine, exacting microscopic surgery.
Perhaps that's the engineer in me. It's continually rewarding, in
that I can generally fix a problem or at least make it a lot better.
Once I graduated, he helped me target the hospitals that would
help me advance my skills and my career. I did my one-year medical internship at New York University Medical Center, then
served my three-year residency under Steven Podos, M.D., Chairman of Ophthalmology at Mount Sinai Hospital in New York
City. Many of the nation's finest ophthalmologists have refined
their skills under Dr. Podos. We are very much the product of his
training.

After my residency, I received a competitive fellowship, known
as the Heed fellowship, which I used to work under two of the
giants of pediatric ophthalmology. I spent six months as appren-
tice to Marshall Parks, M.D., at the Children's National Medical
Center in Washington, D.C., and another six months to Philip
Knapp, M.D., at Columbia-Presbyterian. While in Washington, I
traveled to Johns Hopkins weekly, and in New York, I went to
New York Hospital to learn about tumors in children's eyes. My
fellowship complete, Dr. Knapp—a third generation ophthalmologist—asked me to stay on staff at Columbia in his office. Dr.
Knapp not only knew my work, he knew whom I had studied
with and therefore the quality of expertise I had been privileged to
share. That's how it works in medicine. The "who you know"
part of career building is not just a matter of social status or strategic networking; it indicates the level of knowledge that has been
imparted to you.

This was a radical move, appointing a woman to a hospital
staff that had few women surgical subspecialists. To help me get
started, Dr. Knapp set me up in his office two days a week, without charging me rent. He had put a great deal into my develop-

ment as a doctor and had a stake in my career. This is what I mean when I say that the system is highly personal. During my first years as a surgeon, if I was faced with a difficult operation to perform, Dr. Knapp would often advise me and sometimes sit beside me during surgery, lending insight drawn on his vast experience. Before he died, I sat at his bedside and took notes as he shared with me details of how he handled difficult cases we had not previously discussed. These are the kinds of cases a doctor might see only a handful of times over a lifetime. I keep the papers with the notes from those last sessions in the top drawer of my office desk, and I have referred to them on several occasions. There are patients of mine today who definitely owe their eyesight directly to Dr. Parks's and Dr. Knapp's top-notch skill and expertise.

After a few years working out of Dr. Knapp's office, I moved into my own office at the hospital. Even then, in my first year, I was charged less rent to offset the financial pressure as I built my patient base. That's how it was done: The senior doctors took care of the junior doctors. Today, the economics of medicine has shifted. Astronomical fees for malpractice insurance and rent preclude the kind of breaks that I enjoyed.

But the training and apprenticeship model still holds. I myself now teach second-year medical students how to use our instruments. I train third-years in their one-week ophthalmology course, and I teach eight sections from the entire medical school about pediatric ophthalmology. I advise some medical students, and others approach me with an interest in ophthalmology; some of them even see patients with me. I teach eye residents how to operate.

I am at Columbia-Presbyterian today, a top medical center, because Dr. Parks and Dr. Knapp wanted me there. And they wanted me there because they knew that I had learned from the best.

This is important information for you to know. Where a given physician practices is not random; it's based on personal, professional relationships. A young, less experienced doctor gains his affiliation by the good graces of his peers and elders at a medical institution. To gain hospital privileges, he will have to be vetted by colleagues. The physicians there will know about this new physician from his performance and training pedigree. Frequently in this book, I will stress the wisdom of starting with the medical center in your quest for good medical care. The fact is, if you throw a dart at any major medical center, you're not going to hit a moron; you're going to get somebody near the top of the profession because the powers that be at that institution have chosen him to be there.

HIERARCHY

Medical personnel practice within a clearly defined hierarchy. To the typical medical consumer, all of us look the same. But each of us has a specific expertise and is part of a strict order of command. It is in your interest as a patient to know how this hierarchy works so that you can be sure you're in contact with the appropriate medical care provider and that you deal with this person most effectively.

I find that to explain this hierarchy, military analogies work best. If you walked into any military base, you would notice certain people wearing stripes and a few bearing stars. This immediately clues you into where he or she stands in the pecking order. In medicine, we don't wear stars, but we all know quite well where we are and what that means.

First of all, the change in rank that occurs throughout training is much like that of the military. You start off with the recruits, all of whom go through basic training. The four years of medical school would be the equivalent. There's definitely a boot-camp aspect to medical school: the fierce academic load, long, exhausting hours, an implicit weeding-out process. Once the enlistees emerge triumphant from initial training, they splinter off into military specialties within their branch; similarly, newly minted doctors go on to residencies in the basic fields of medicine. The enlistees divide up into tank gunners, fliers, etc; in medicine, these would be specialties—the area of practice within the broader category. Finally, some would move into special elite groups, like the Navy Seals or Green Berets. Likewise, some subspecialists spend additional fellowship years training in highly specialized areas of treatment and diagnosis, such as pediatric hematology and neuropsychiatry.

Just where a doctor fits in this structure determines what he does and what others will ask of him. Say a certain soldier is known to be a super marksman. He'll be first to be called when a sharp eye is needed, but no one will expect him to be an expert flier. Similarly, you are unlikely to chase down an orthopedist to insert a catheter. He will be able to do it, but it's not the best use of his time. Everyone has an area of expertise. Within the larger group, different people will be put forward in different situations. Everybody is important to the larger task. Nurses are like the flight crew in the air force. The equipment that they manage has to be in perfect working order or everything fails; their scrutiny of patient needs keeps physicians informed. What they do is crucial, even if you don't see it.

People on the inside understand the division of labor, the "who does what" and "who can say what to whom." This hierarchy is communicated to others within the system in ways that might go right over an outsider's head. In a study, officers and enlisted men were all put in their underwear. Still, a group of recruits questioned knew exactly who was who. The same holds true for medicine. In the operating room, for example, a patient, seeing nothing more than a sea of green or blue scrub outfits, would be unsure who is going to be operating on him and who is support staff. But ask anyone in the operating room (OR) and they'll know. In observing the way medical people act around each other, you can figure it out, too. When one person walks into a room, and everyone else snaps to attention, that suggests that the newcomer is near the top of the pyramid of expertise. What we now refer to as the OR used to be called the "surgical theater," an appropriate name since everyone in the room has a clearly defined role to play.

In the course of treatment, a patient can meet a generalist and a supersubspecialist and not know whom they're dealing with. Therefore they may waste questions or ask questions outside of a person's expertise. You could end up asking the same question three times. The questions you ask need to be within the context of that person's role. You'll get better care because you can zip up and down the line of command.

Let me give you an example from my own field. I am a child's eye specialist. Any ophthalmologist can do an eye exam, but my exams are tailored to a child. I am probably more familiar with eye problems unique to children or common among children than, say, a general ophthalmologist. Similarly, I could do an adult eye exam. But a general ophthalmologist would probably be better suited to do that.

Recently, I was examining a young boy and noticed that he was having trouble hearing me. When I pointed this out to his mother, she said that his hearing had been tested in the pediatrician's office and was found to be okay. She went on to explain that he had gone to the pediatrician because of a cough; it was determined that the cough was psychosomatic because it tended to kick up when school started.

A bell went off in my head, and I thought, a cold—possibly asthma. Based on my judgment and twenty years' experience working with kids, I said, "I think you have a chronic problem." I'm a vision specialist; I am not an expert on hearing, but I knew enough to know that something might be wrong. I suggested that the boy see a pediatric ear, nose, and throat (ENT) specialist, whose perspective may be different from the child's pediatrician's. The specialist found that the child had cold-induced asthma (cold season, incidentally, coincides with the start of school), and a CT scan revealed that the boy also suffered from sinus problems. With the appropriate medication, his cough disappeared, his sinuses were cleared, and his hearing improved.

The pediatrician who had dismissed the boy's cough as psychosomatic didn't do harm or mistreat the problem; the family had simply reached the limit of his expertise. He could do no more for his patient. With my specialization, I see a subgroup of disorders in different configurations, and from my particular perspective, I saw this child's problem in a different context.

The lesson to be learned here is when you've been checked out and you have a lingering feeling that something is still wrong, pursue it. Go to the next level of expertise. Ideally, the pediatrician should have referred the child to a specialist, but he didn't. Rather than follow their instincts and pursue more specialized diagnoses, the family was simply reassured by what the pediatrician said.

As a patient or the parent of a patient, you need to know the context for the medical visit at hand. You're not going to go to a pizza place and ask for filet mignon; you won't expect something fabulous there. Your expectations of each person's role have to be reasonable.

The big picture, the larger framework of medical specialization, can be confusing and overwhelming. It can all look the same—a big blur of white coats, intimidating degrees, and cryptic abbreviations attached to unfamiliar names. When you can start to see the patterns, though, it becomes a lot clearer. And that knowledge can help guide you through your own medical encounters.

PROFESSIONAL RESPECT

A key unwritten rule among physicians is not to step on one another's toes. One reflection of this is the reluctance to criticize another doctor. Some people get angry with us because they believe that we're protecting one another. While there is some truth to that, it is far more complicated than the notion of doctors closing ranks to cover up for one of their own. The reality is that, as a physician, you really don't know what *you* would have done in the same situation. This is partly because you can never really know what it's like to be in another's shoes, and partly because the case as presented may not be exactly how it was. The Monday-morning quarterbacking sessions that you might see on the television show *ER* can never re-create what actually happened. It's always easy to work a case over when you're sitting with your cup of coffee and a donut, but when you're rushing between ten rooms and people are dying in front of you, it's different. Criticizing another doctor doesn't help anybody. And your criticism may be unfounded because you don't have all the facts.

Still, there are diplomatic ways to convey doubts about another doctor's clinical prowess. I learned how physicians communicate their misgivings through the case of a patient I care dearly about, my mother. When I was a second-year medical student, my mother had a medical problem. Her doctor was sending her to another doctor in the same practice for a diagnostic procedure. By coincidence, we had recently had a lecture on that particular syndrome, and something about her recommended treatment didn't sound right to me.

I approached my professor after class and told him about my mother and what they wanted to do. His eyes widened and he said, "Really?" I said, "Yes, but you had said something else." I kept waiting for him to contradict the doctor, but he didn't. He did say that my mother should get a second opinion outside of the same group practice. In this way he let me know that the treatment was wrong, suggested an appropriate next step, and protected my mother from an unnecessary procedure—all this without criticizing my mother's care. In so doing, he demonstrated to me how to be an elegant physician.

I reached my mother by phone and urged her to forgo the test, but, alas, it had already been done. Eventually, she went elsewhere to deal with her problem. I tucked this experience away in my memory because I found it unsettling. I didn't understand its import until much later. My professor was used to seeing improprieties. In fact, he indicated to me that she should have gone to another physician. But he had responded as a gentleman. It wasn't that he didn't care about me or what happened to my mother, but it wasn't for him to say that this was a bad doctor. All he could know was that the doctor seemed to be using poor judgment. But we don't say these things, you understand. "Go to another doctor" is the answer.

Another means of showing respect for fellow physicians is respecting another physician's clinical role. I make sure not to get in the position of translating what another doctor says. If a patient that has been referred to me says that she hears one thing from Dr. X and a different thing from Dr. Y, I might explain to the patient that we all speak differently. I would then explain my variation until the patient had no further questions.

In other instances, I would make sure not go over the referring physician's head to deliver a diagnosis. I will tell them about my "eye findings" from the examination. However, I would not be comfortable making any broader conclusions about what that means for a patient's health. If people press me—and, being hungry for information, they sometimes do—I say, "Look, you have too many people telling you things. I will give my information to your primary care physician, who can give you the larger picture." I will then call the primary doctor so he or she can put it into a "total body" context, with my examination as one puzzle piece. It is important that a patient hears about his or her status in one voice, and the best spokesperson is the primary physician, even when that physician has encouraged the patient to consult a specialist. From my perspective as a pediatric eye specialist, I may see the situation one way. But the physician who has the overview, who knows more about the patient's overall medical condition, may choose to see information another way.

CERTIFICATION

The medical community maintains a strict credentialing system. This is the quality control for physicians. Those letters after the M.D. on a doctor's stationery and the framed diplomas on the wall tell you the credentials he or she has acquired and which organizations have given their stamp of approval to that physician. The certification process gives medical consumers a great deal of information about prospective physicians—but most people don't know how to interpret the data. In medicine, as in everything else, there is never a guarantee. It's all percentage. The certification system tells you how many hoops a physician has jumped through, and you want to know that your physician has jumped through as many hoops as possible within his or her expertise.

To give you a sense of how physicians get checked out, I will tell you which hoops I've had to jump through. After the second year of medical school, I took a full two-day examination, Part I (of three) of the National Board Examination. In some medical schools, entry into the third year is contingent on passing this exam. I took Part II, which can be taken either at the end of the third year or during the fourth year, during my third year. And I took Part III toward the end of my internship, the year of clinical immersion after medical school. Although I had received my M.D. the previous spring, I became licensed to practice only after passing all three parts *and* applying to New York State to validate my credentials.

After my residency, in the middle of my fellowship year, I sat for a half-day written Board Examination in Ophthalmology. After receiving a pass (nearly a quarter of those who take it fail), I qualified to take a two-day oral exam in seven sections the next fall. Upon passing the oral exam I became board-certified by the

American Board of Ophthalmology. After my fellowship, I applied to the American Association of Pediatric Ophthalmology and Strabismus (AAPOS). To pass this hurdle, I had to submit written recommendations from my fellowship mentors, documentation of an AAPOS-approved fellowship, licenses, and transcripts.

These credentials situate me quite specifically in the world of medicine. I am a physician (M.D.) licensed in the state of New York. I have been certified by the American Board of Ophthalmology. (Another way of saying this is that I am a fellow of the American Board of Ophthalmology.) I belong to the organization that governs my subspecialty, AAPOS. After being in practice for a few years *and* performing a specified number of surgeries, I became a fellow of the American College of Surgeons (FACS). Later I became a fellow of the American Association of Pediatrics (FAAP), as befits my subspecialty of Pediatric Ophthalmology.

On the academic side, I am a faculty member of the Columbia University College of Physicians and Surgeons and an associate professor of Ophthalmology in the Department of Ophthalmology and an associate professor of Pediatrics in the Department of Pediatrics of the Columbia-Presbyterian Medical Center.

Some physicians are listed as "board-eligible" or "active candidates for the board." Such doctors are licensed by the state to practice medicine but do not have board certification. This could be because they are in just their first or second year of practice and have not completed their training. Or they may have applied for board certification and failed part of the test. (Candidates can take the examination three times.) If a board-eligible doctor is thirty years old, that's okay. If he or she is fifty, I'd wonder.

Patients are at a disadvantage when they don't understand the certification process and categories. I know a couple, both quite prominent in their professions, who had to amend arrangements for their small daughter's medical care because of this disadvantage. Their three-year-old girl needed treatment for a heart condition. Their physician referred them to a pediatric cardiologist, who recommended surgery. They asked around about heart surgeons and were set to go with a well-regarded *adult* cardiac surgeon who had treated a contemporary of theirs. I pointed out to them that they needed a *pediatric* heart surgeon to operate on their child. You want someone trained in and accustomed to operating on little bodies. My friends hadn't known that such a person existed; they thought that consulting the pediatric cardiologist was enough. Before you can know what you want, you have to know what's out there.

THE DOCTOR "PERSONALITY"

People often make assumptions about doctors' personalities. On the one hand, people expect doctors to be both invulnerable and infallible, so they become enraged if a physician betrays any doubt or weakness. On the other hand, people complain about physicians being "cold" or "aloof," thinking it means they don't care.

You need to understand that doctors are trained to manage their emotions so that they can do their work. One of the things they teach us in medical school is that terrible things will happen to your patients. However, if you're crying your eyes out about a bad outcome, you won't be able to help the next ten patients who need your care. You still have to function. That's the bottom line. But that very ability to keep yourself functioning may be interpreted as not caring. The point is that, as a doctor, you are trained to put those feelings on the back burner so that you don't sell your other patients short.

There is a certain war-zone mentality that you learn to adopt. As a surgeon, for example, you may have to make a decision about what or how much to cut. You don't have time to look up five references in the library. You have to make the decision *now*. Some of these will be low-level decisions, but even these will be intimidating at first. In time you master those kinds of decisions and learn to face the harder challenges. People say of surgeons, "They just want to operate." We feel unfairly tarnished by this. The fact is that surgeons are highly opinionated. We believe in what we do. That's a requirement of the job. We think that what we're offering is the best option available.

Similarly, a lot of people think that oncologists are cold fish. But here you have someone who has to deliver a difficult cancer diagnosis and then immediately move on to evaluate the next patient. He or she has to carry that pain inside, but not be overwhelmed by it. Too many people are counting on his or her care.

CHAPTER TWO

The Medical Center:
Your Most Important Choice

T HE MOST SIGNIFICANT DECISION you make in setting up your medical care is choosing a hospital or medical center. If that surprises you, you're not alone. Most people consider the hospital secondary to the physician. After all, the physician is the one who tends to *you*. The hospital is seen simply as the backdrop, the setting for your physician's care. But a smart medical consumer will zero in on the hospital. One reason is that all hospitals are not created equal. Another is that once you've chosen a hospital, you're well on your way to getting your personal medical care system in place.

The old model of medical care was based on the sole-proprietor small business; a doctor ran a kind of Mom-and-Pop operation. Today, however, doctors function as part of a larger organization. When in search of a treatment or diagnosis, rarely do you consult and receive care from just one doctor. As a consumer, you need to think in terms of the larger organization—in terms of the doctors connected to your primary physician—and choose on the basis of the quality and availability of resources, for that one choice will determine every other aspect of your health care. Learn what you can about your hospital options. Before you put your toe in the water, it's best to figure out what kind of pond you're dealing with.

Addressing the hospital question first helps you keep the big picture in mind. Then, once you're hooked into the hospital, you can find an appropriate physician because many physicians will serve at that hospital. When you work with a doctor, you are really working with a team of doctors—a team of generalists, specialists, and subspecialists continually working together through consultation and referral. The smart strategy is to pick the team and then choose the player. Think of the Yankees in baseball. All the players are good. Some are better than others, of course, but deciding to put a Yankee on the field gives you a certain guarantee of quality. It's much the same way in medicine. It's not easy to join a hospital's rank. A doctor can't just waltz up and say, "I want to practice medicine here"; he or she has to be chosen. So if you pick a good team—a good hospital—the institution has done a good amount of the sifting through for you.

No doctor works in a vacuum, so you want to know your doctor has good teammates. Even the simplest exam may require lab tests or X-rays, which means that other medical personnel are already part of your care. As a colleague of mine noted, we rarely see a patient without ordering something or interacting at least informally with someone else. The competence, timeliness, and judgment of these "invisible" doctors can have a great impact on the treatment you get, without your necessarily knowing it. Although you did not select these other medical professionals individually, you have de facto selected them by choosing a particular institution.

Every patient benefits from the connections between physicians that evolve over time. As a doctor in a hospital, I become used to interacting with other affiliated physicians. The importance of such working relationships may not be apparent to the outside. For example, let's say I call a pulmonary specialist at my medical center and say, "I have a patient I would like you to see."

He would snap to attention. Why? Not because he's doing me a favor, but because he knows that I rarely call him. He will remember that the last time I called him on a patient's behalf, it was serious. And of course it's reciprocal. I'll listen when he calls me. Collegial relationships like this are part of an institution's package.

The hospital also serves as a base for an entire referral network. When you need a specialist, you don't want to be flipping idly through the yellow pages. In any hospital, there are established referral patterns that have achieved prior results. Sure, you can choose your own specialists, but there's a lot to be said for going with a specialist whom your primary care physician is used to working with and knows will treat you well.

What you are looking for in a hospital is internal quality control. A hospital will allow only people with a certain level of credentials to get on staff. You want to know that the hospital you go to has a level of quality control that's extremely rigorous and goes across all the specialties. It's a lot like going to a hotel: If you go to a Four Seasons Hotel, you're assured that all the services are good and that everyone who serves you is professional, so you don't need to worry about each and every detail. You want some sense of quality because, with any hospital, you're not just getting your doctor; you're getting everything and everybody else.

But first you need to know what kind of hospitals are out there.

DIFFERENT TYPES OF HOSPITALS

The Joint Commission of American Hospitals certifies hospitals on three levels: tertiary, secondary, and primary. In general, tertiary refers to the major medical centers, secondary to good community hospitals, and primary to small rural hospitals. What the differences mean to your actual care may not be immediately evident. Let's look at what you get.

TERTIARY MEDICAL CENTERS

These are the names you've heard: Columbia-Presbyterian Medical Center, UCLA, Massachusetts General, Washington University, Baylor Medical Center, Mayo Clinic, Johns Hopkins. These are full-service, major medical centers. To carry the hotel analogy a bit further, these are the luxury hotels of the hospital world; every possible need has been anticipated. During a stay at the Ritz, you can call room service at 3:00 A.M. and order fois gras, a cheeseburger, or whatever strikes your fancy. Services are that extensive: No matter what you want, they have it when you need it. You may not know in advance that you want it, and that's the point. The hospital equivalent of the Ritz has a helipad, a full surgical team (doctors, an anesthesiologist, and specialized nurses) not merely "available" but actually ready to take care of you, and every specialist and subspecialist known to man. There are not just neurosurgeons, but neurosurgeons who do backs, neurosurgeons who do tumors inside the head, neurosurgeons who work with seizures. There are ENT (ear, nose, and throat) people who specialize in ears, who specialize in noses, who specialize in cancer, and so on. Among the pediatric staff, there's likely to be an entire children's surgical specialty group, with pediatric surgical subspecialists in ophthalmology, orthopedics, neurosurgery, cardiology, ENT, urology, and pathology, plus a squadron of general surgeons.

Sometimes you need all this, sometimes you don't. But what you're getting at a major medical center is predictability in circumstances that may be unpredictable. Whatever you come in with, they've seen it before. That's important. If, for example, you are anticipating a complicated delivery, the hospital would have an obstetrician, a pediatric neonatologist, and an anesthesiologist or two waiting in the wings to address any problems. And that's only the personnel you know about.

A hospital is all about the people who staff it. It's not just about a pretty place or equipment. Looks may be deceiving.

Many less-than-the-Four-Seasons hospitals are well tended and beautiful. Likewise, a fine major medical center may have dingy offices or hallways. But when you get down to the issue of what's being done for you, don't reject an old physical plant. Because it's not the machines that are important, but the people who run them.

Here is the story of someone who allowed himself to be swayed by the niceties of a lesser place, to his detriment:

John, a family friend and the former CEO of a large financial company, had a complicated neck problem. He was from New York but now lived on the west coast of Florida. He saw a local physician, whose immediate response was, "Go up north and see a neurosurgeon." In New York, he gathered opinions from several good physicians, and it looked as if the surgery was all set. Then he got a call from his nephew in Florida, a physician administrator for a small community hospital (note: beware of well-meaning relatives) who said, "I've got a great hospital down here," meaning Florida's *east* coast. "I will take good care of you in my hospital. Come here." When I heard about this, I told John, "No, the place is too small. The surgery should be done in a place where they regularly do this kind of thing. If it were my neck, I'd go north."

I could see no advantage to having the surgery in eastern Florida. Since it was an hour's flight away, his wife would still have to camp out. And while the orthopedist may have been every bit as wonderful as they said, an operation like this should be done by an experienced neurosurgeon. The smaller hospital would have only a general anesthesiologist rather than a neuro-anesthesiologist. And the surgery was especially complicated because the incision would need to be made in the front. I was nervous about this.

The day of the surgery, I got a call from my mother: "The anesthesia went fine, but the surgeon put his finger through John's esophagus (swallowing tube)." "[Expletive deleted]," I said. The plan now was to wait two weeks and attempt the surgery again.

"What? Go back there?" I said to John when I talked to him later.

"They were so nice," he said. "The surgeon was so apologetic about what happened."

Of course he was apologetic—he was no doubt mortified, if not terrified of a malpractice suit, and, as a diligent physician, quite concerned. Meanwhile, I asked an orthopedist colleague if this kind of thing happened often. He said, "I know it's a rare complication." I pressed him: "Actually, I never saw it in training or heard of it happening anywhere during that time."

When John went home to recover, his local doctor urged him to rethink his plan, saying, "Will you please go to a larger medical center? Look what almost happened to you!"

John finally agreed to go to New York and had a pre-operative meeting with the anesthesiologist, who asked detailed questions about his medical history, including a previous heart attack. "They never asked me these questions before," he said. "I've never seen anyone so thorough in my life!" Well, this was a neuro-anesthesiologist. At this point, however, the surgery was twice as hard because it was a redo. Nevertheless, because of the surgeon's competency and experience with the exact procedure, the operation was a success. But now John is angry because his neck hurts. Of course his neck hurts—he had two surgeries!

This wasn't a disaster, this was a near-disaster. And a warning.

What you want from a hospital is staff with expertise and judgment. You want people who have seen what you have as well as variations of what you have so they see the patterns and understand how it all fits together diagnostically. You want to be prepared for every contingency. In a top-notch hospital, at any given time you have operating rooms on full alert like the F-16 pilots who were flying over my house for a couple of months after September 11, making me feel very nice and secure. In fact, they lulled me to sleep. They were flying over the Hudson between Manhattan and a nuclear plant not far away, and they were protecting us from any mishaps or attacks. It was really nice to hear those guys. I never said hello to them. I never even waved. The same is true at the hospital. You don't have to acknowledge everyone who's there to protect you, but it's nice to know they're there.

SECONDARY MEDICAL CENTERS

Many fine local hospitals serve their communities well. They are generally very good at basic care. Community hospitals are often easier to get to and more user-friendly. You can have excellent results because there are many highly competent physicians and staff who have trained at top-tier medical centers and now work in the community hospitals. Areas near major cities in particular will have highly skilled subspecialists with good training and experience. While you can get basic care in the tertiary medical center, it's fine to go locally, too. It's a lower-stress option. You can park down the street, pick your kids up from nursery school on the way home, and you don't have to set aside a whole day for your appointment.

If you're considering surgery and other treatments at a secondary hospital, make sure they perform the surgery you need in some kind of volume. One physician friend in upstate New York needed coronary artery bypass surgery and a valve replacement. This is an old-fashioned family doctor kind of guy who never missed a day of work because of illness, and his family was thinking of getting him into one of the top centers known for bypass surgery. But he decided to stay in Schenectady and have the surgery in the hospital where he had seen patients his entire career. He had interviewed the surgeon and saw that the numbers were good. (Note that he did his homework even though he was a colleague.) Because his particular situation was at the low end of the complication scale, and because he knew the hospital and staff and felt comfortable there, he decided that the benefits of staying local outweighed the advantages of going to a major medical center. It was a small enough place that he wouldn't be just another cog in the wheel. Also, it would be easier for his family to visit and, in the postoperative period, to care for him. All

AFFILIATE HOSPITALS

A lot of major urban medical centers are sending groups of M.D.s to suburbs. This is potentially a good development, a way of spreading the wealth geographically. For example, some physicians at Columbia-Presbyterian's Babies Hospital spend part of their time at fine regional hospitals. The best scenario is when the medical center and the peripheral hospital work out a symbiotic relationship. Valley Hospital in New Jersey, for instance, has a cadre of excellent subspecialists because the standard for doctors on staff is very high. They knew they needed certain doctors, but they knew that the volume couldn't completely support such specialists' practices. So they created a scenario where the physicians could do routine cases there and bring more complicated cases where they needed additional support back to the city. Physicians would end up splitting their surgery practices: Monday in the suburbs, Tuesday in the city, etc. The doctors are hopping around, deciding where best to treat each patient. The presence of academically high-qualified physicians at a peripheral institution raises the level of care at that institution. This is becoming a widespread model for care.

This kind of outreach has led to some confusion, however. Be aware that the presence of a fine institution's name doesn't guarantee that you're getting that institution's care. Theoretically, an affiliate hospital will represent the same fine training and retain the same staff protocols as the home institution. But sometimes there is no more than a paper affiliation, perhaps involving the rental of space. Here's how to sort it out: Check the department roster of the main hospital to see if the physician in question is listed on the staff. The hospital will be able to provide you with the information you need to find out the physician's degree of affiliation and level of credentials.

surgery begins with the surgery and *only ends weeks later with the patient's recovery*. With major surgery, this can be a very bumpy ride, and as disruptive as the operation itself.

Increasingly, hospitals are part of a complicated, interlocking system that works to deliver the optimal level of care. When a local hospital doesn't have the appropriate subspecialist, they send the patient to the medical center. Otherwise, they keep the patient locally and give him very fine treatment. Doctors now participating in these feeder systems have honed successful working relationships with fellow physicians and specialists, so you can feel confident that they're placing you in capable hands.

Typically, a local hospital will have an emergency room with a licensed emergency specialist and some very fine nurses who function like resident doctors. But it might not have a full set of pediatric equipment in the ER. And, unlike major medical centers, it doesn't have resident doctors and would have to call in experts for anything out of the ordinary. That's fine for most things. But at a major medical center, it would all be there already.

Ideally, this is how the different levels of hospitals work together. On Christmas Eve, someone I knew had a heart attack and went to a very tiny community hospital in Dobbs Ferry, New York. That night somebody very smart was moonlighting in the emergency room. He said, "We can't take care of this problem. You need to go to the medical center now." He shipped the patient out because, as an emergency room doctor, he knew that he didn't have the facilities or the people, all of which was exacerbated by the bad timing of Christmas Eve. The man went down to Montefiore Hospital in the Bronx via ambulance, and at midnight they did an angioplasty that saved his life. It went smoothly because Dobbs Ferry got on the phone with Montefiore and said, "We've got one for you. He's coming." That conversation made the whole thing happen.

These smaller and midsized hospitals provide a very important function for the community. For your own medical care, you can start locally and work your way up the specialty ladder and into the tertiary medical center if you need to. Or, you can start at the bigger place so you can develop a relationship with the institution and the people there. But the *most important thing* is to get in the system.

PRIMARY MEDICAL CENTERS

A rural hospital is generally chosen by geographical default. You're there because you live in a rural area or because you happen to be there when you fall ill or become injured. Usually, what you're dealing with is nice people, lesser facilities. You can get very good care, particularly for routine problems. The fact is that physicians in rural hospitals do not have the volume or assortment of patients needed to be up on all aspects of medicine. People there tend to be jacks-of-all-trades. Also, since the pool is much smaller, you will not have as great a choice of whom to consult. You can be lucky and find a gem of a doctor. But as a rule, the more choice you have, the more likely you are to find someone good. However, small rural hospitals are usually good about transferring patients to larger centers if they lack the facilities for their care, often airlifting people out to a regional trauma center. Patients who have chronic diseases can drive to larger cities in the region for more specialized care.

EMERGENCIES: NEVER ASSUME THEY'RE SIMPLE

A smaller hospital's emergency room may be fine for straightforward problems. Unfortunately, you can't always assume that a problem is straightforward. For example, one Sunday afternoon, a neighbor's son came running over to our house screaming: His dad had slashed his finger in the kitchen as he was removing a knife from the dishwasher. I wasn't sure exactly what we were dealing with, but he had certainly done a good job on himself. Hands are

STICK WITH THE SAME MEDICAL INSTITUTION THROUGHOUT A COURSE OF TREATMENT

A friend's uncle needed complicated surgery for a rare abdominal tumor. His internist put him in touch with a truly superlative general surgeon at Columbia-Presbyterian, probably one of the few in the country who had dealt with this unusual and inaccessible cancer. The surgery—an eight-hour procedure—was a success, and the man went home to recover. He was doing well until, two weeks later, he became nauseated and dizzy. It was late at night. His wife drove him to the local emergency room and he was admitted to the hospital for several days. He was treated for pancreatitis, an irritation of the pancreas, and an infection near the incision, and then returned home.

I would have urged him to return to Columbia-Presbyterian, only five minutes further from his house. Here's why: When there's a complication after surgery, the surgeon is the person most likely to know what the problem is. The surgeon may have seen a similar complication or may have a sense of what might go wrong in the follow-up period. Also, as a surgeon, it's easier to fix your own complications. Another operation (referred to as a "re-op") or follow-up treatment may be necessary, and the person who performed the surgery needs to be in on it. But it was late at night and they were scared. They thought, "Well, it's not related to the surgery. Let's go to our regular place." First, it probably *is* related to the surgery. And now there's a big disconnect between the patient and the person who knows most about his situation—the surgeon.

When you're dealing with follow-up problems, the best way to cover your bases is to stay with the same hospital. It is an insurance measure you can take to avoid disaster. And by this I mean *your* disaster—that's all that you care about. They could have called their surgeon when he didn't feel well. Postoperative care *is* part of the surgery. You are *not* bothering your doctor about it—and if so, too bad—for this is what it means to take **ca**re of you. Surgery may begin when you enter the operating room but it doesn't end when you leave.

complicated; there are a lot of tendons. This could be a really major problem, or fairly easily treated. You don't know—it all looks the same at first. The poor guy was turning white, not in a position to make any decisions. He said, "You tell me what to do."

I called the chief hand surgeon at Columbia and described the situation. He told me to take my friend to the emergency room at the local hospital. "Get him treated," he said. "He can come and see me afterward." The local hospital happened to be extremely busy. My friend wasn't dying, so his case was placed on the back burner. I told the person checking in with us that I wanted a plastic surgeon to see him. It took an hour and a half for the guy to come down from northern Westchester. We had no idea that he'd be coming so far. It turned out that, in slicing his finger nearly to the bone, he had cut a tendon. The plastic surgeon repaired it partially in the ER, then my friend saw a good hand surgeon.

I reported this to Columbia's chief hand surgeon, who said that he would have done it in an operating room instead of the emergency room. The OR is a more controlled environment; you can use a microscope, and there are more options for regional anesthesia. The ER doctor used only local anesthesia, which numbed the hand. In an operating room, an anesthesiologist could have used an arm block or put the patient to sleep. Had I brought my friend to Columbia-Presbyterian instead of the local hospital, this is what would have happened: The emergency room would have called the surgery resident. The resident, in turn, would have called the fellow in hand surgery. The fellow would have evaluated the patient and made a judgment in consultation with a senior hand surgeon by phone. There was nothing wrong with the care my friend received and he was okay, but I will not make that mistake again. The next time there is any question, I am going into the city to the bigger hospital.

The tough part about emergencies is that you need to make a decision at a time when you're least able to do so rationally. All the more reason for you to understand the kinds of choices that you have ahead of time. Here's where I did some learning in the trenches:

My twelve-year-old daughter was playing tennis when she tripped and split her chin open. She was driven back to our house and arrived screaming with blood spilling down her shirt. (Note: She should have immediately been taken to the emergency room, and I would have met her there.)

Anyway, she was delivered bleeding and screaming to my front door. Now, when your child is screaming, you do not think clearly. There are no exceptions to this. I called the pediatrician, asked for a list of good local plastic surgeons, and took my daughter to the emergency room at our local community hospital, which I knew was good. (Another note: *Before* you're in a crisis, make sure that you know how to get to your local emergency room, whether there are one-way streets to navigate, etc. We ended up driving around for ten extremely long minutes because, unbeknownst to us, the entrance to the ER had been moved!) I asked the emergency staff person to call in a plastic surgeon. After forty-five minutes and no plastic surgeon (it's a Saturday and one guy's at a wedding, another's out of town), they urge us to let the ER doctor take care of the chin.

I went out into the waiting room and called Columbia-Presbyterian to see if anyone there was available. I knew the emergency doctors were competent, but I also knew that I wanted a board-certified plastic surgeon to take care of my daughter's injury. It wasn't that the ER doctors weren't good. It was that I knew the percentages were better with the board-certified professional. I didn't want to find this out the hard way: I wanted predictability. The *board-certified* part was my personal insurance policy. The nurse came out and said how wonderful the ER doctor was and that I should let him do it. By now I was completely stressed. I hated to be confrontational at a moment like this, but at the same time I knew what I wanted for my daughter. I said, "We're getting the board-certified person or

I'm leaving." To her credit, the nurse said she understood and let me be.

The point I want to make here is that if you're not comfortable with a proposed course of action, you don't have to say yes. People are often afraid to say no, but unless it's truly a life-threatening situation—like acute appendicitis—you don't have to accept treatment you don't want. It is within your right to ask for the higher-level professional. If you don't have days and weeks to find other options, you may have minutes or hours. In this case, I had a few hours in which to maneuver, and I knew that you have eight hours to sew up an incision. (After eight hours, it's too late to sew up a laceration neatly due to infection and certain properties of healing.) By this time, my daughter had stopped bleeding and calmed down. The bottom line then for me was this: I didn't want to have her stitched up and then find out that it would have been done better by someone more experienced.

By now I had become an inconvenience to the emergency room staff and they wanted us treated and out of there. They found us a fine, board-certified plastic surgeon—number five on their calling list, not because he wasn't good, but because of the way the rotations fell—and he did a fine job. He had to close the wound in three levels because it was split down to the bone. One couldn't have known how deep it was until the process was underway. It's hard to evaluate a wound until you really inspect it. And that's something you can't do as a bystander, relative, or nontreating physician.

A REAL TOUGH CASE

It takes enormous presence of mind to question medical treatment during an emergency. But having the fortitude to evaluate the level of care, even to the point of making changes if necessary, can make a great difference in the outcome. One situation, in which parents made a difficult but ultimately life-saving decision for their child in the aftermath of a car wreck, has always stayed with me.

Several years back, a group of high school seniors in our town were tooling down a highway at 3 A.M. and hit a tree. The driver was killed instantly. A friend's daughter, in the back-middle seat, broke her arm; she got off easy. One young man ruptured his aorta. He was brought to the county medical center, where it took two operations to successfully sew up his the rupture.

One girl had an upper body injury. She was also brought to the county medical center, but her parents were uncomfortable and had her transferred to a pediatric orthopedist at Columbia-Presbyterian. After she had been there two days, the orthopedist realized that her neck was extremely destabilized. If you look at the spinal area, the disks of your back are lined up on a pole. After this girl's injury, the pole was broken in one place. What this meant was that one of the disks in her upper neck was unhinged, and would sooner or later slide forward and cut her spinal cord. If this had been allowed to happen, she would instantly have become a quadriplegic.

The staff at the county medical center had tried to discourage the parents from taking their daughter to another hospital. "What's wrong? We're doing fine," they said. However, the parents knew that there was a higher level of expertise and specialization in a children's hospital, so they overrode the system. The first place—which called itself a medical center but was not in fact a high-quality place—had missed a serious problem. Because of the second orthopedist's expertise, he found the problem and was able to address it in a timely way. The young woman will have lifelong problems as a result of this injury, but she's not bound to a wheelchair. The parents were right. You don't want to be right. But it's better than the alternative.

CHOOSING THE HOSPITAL THAT'S RIGHT FOR YOU

Here are some tips for selecting a hospital to be the cornerstone of your care:

Read its report card. The first thing you want to do is establish that the hospital is good. That sounds obvious. But most people don't know that straightforward information about a hospital's quality is readily available. All hospitals are required to be licensed, and every licensed hospital receives regular accreditation from the Joint Commission of American Hospitals (JCAH) in which they are graded in different areas. The accreditation report is publicly available. You can call the hospital administrator's office and ask what their JCAH rating is. Some hospitals are on probation. Others have really good grades. In either case, you want to know.

Ask what subspecialists it has. If only two are named, I wouldn't go to that hospital. The number of specialists at an institution suggests how often there's a need for a specialist and therefore the hospital's experience in a given area. Generalists are important. But you need to have other specialties represented, or at least in the loop.

Find out who staffs the emergency room. Don't assume anything. Is the ER licensed as an emergency room? Emergency medicine is now a medical specialty; is there someone specialized in emergency medicine who staffs it, or do they use a rotating group of doctors from the staff? Avoid the latter, if you have a choice.

Ask if there is a pediatric emergency room. If there is, find out if it is staffed by a board-certified ER doctor who specializes in pediatrics. Not every emergency room has equipment sized for children, such as special tubes and surgical tools.

Ask if it is a designated trauma center. By design, such centers are spread out all over the country. It suggests a higher degree of expertise because a trauma center is equipped to deal with everything. Increasingly, hospitals are beginning to collaborate by designating one hospital in an area a trauma center so that, in a particular region, all the police or emergency workers will naturally go to the same place. Because resources have been pooled, patients get extremely fine care. With increased volume, rare problems become routine. The medical staff becomes quite experienced, and therefore they function at a high level. If you do the same thing ten times a month, you're better at it than if you only do it once a year. If you spread out the trauma cases among several hospitals, you'll wind up with a doctor who hasn't seen a punctured lung since perhaps last month. With a regional trauma center, the doctor may be seeing three a day.

Familiarize yourself with its role in the vertical hierarchy. If you're looking at a small hospital, you will want to know where the institution fits into the vertical hierarchy. You want to know what hospital it feeds into should the need for more specialized care arise. You may decide to get basic care at the small local hospital and then move up to a larger hospital for problems demanding greater expertise.

Find out if it is affiliated with a medical school. If so, which one? This is good to know. In general, the more complicated cases get fed to hospitals affiliated with medical schools. This is a function of the apprenticeship hierarchy. Simply knowing that a hospital is affiliated with a medical school gives you important information. In order to support medical training, a hospital needs a very diverse staff. The institution has to be able to teach students everything they're supposed to know. This is strictly controlled by medical school accreditation. With a medical school affiliation, you have residents and fellows, the whole shebang. This training is superimposed on the tertiary medical model, so that the physicians are interacting on a very high level of complexity and specialization.

Seek out the hospital with the expertise you need. If you're looking for a specific area of expertise, find out who has it. For example, in New York City, New York Hospital has the best burn unit. The other medical institutions in the city have pretty much deferred to New York Hospital for serious burn cases so that severe burn problems all get taken there. This doesn't mean that other hospitals can't treat a burn. But burn treatment is highly esoteric and labor intensive, requiring an extended, highly trained staff.

New York Hospital became so good at it that it was better to support their effort than to try to compete. It would have been impossible to maintain two equal burn units with the same high-level, specialized staff, and care couldn't be as good in the lesser one.

Investigate its claims. If a hospital claims expertise, find out how deep it goes. In many geographical areas, hospitals have tried to buy segments of the medical market. For example, one local hospital may advertise the best cardiac center in the region. This may mean that they have hired one really fine specialist and given him or her funds to buy staff and equipment. The cardiac care may be good, but there may not be an equivalent neurosurgeon down the hall, and anesthesia and ICU back-up may be lacking.

Keep your priorities straight. Some of the outlying hospitals have built up expertise in one area. Take, for instance, some of the newer cardiac and cancer centers. These are real money-makers. They also tend to be patient-centered: There's plush carpeting, the nurses are nice, you get a cup of coffee and—here's the pay-off—you get fine care because they bought a superb physician from a major medical center. There is nothing wrong with that. However, you have to evaluate the entire picture—not just the big shot, but the other associated doctors and staff. This is hard to do when you're hurting; you want to be at a place that's nice to you, and it all looks good. *But it's the people who matter, not the carpeting.*

Ask around. Find out where your friends have gotten good care. If you have a choice of local hospitals, ask people which they like best. If you know a nurse or doctor that you can ask, you'll get a better answer.

CHAPTER THREE

Getting the Best from Your Primary Care Doctor

⟋⟍

I N ALL MEDICAL MATTERS, your primary care physician—an internist, a general practitioner, or, for a child, a pediatrician— is the linchpin: the medical professional who holds everything together. The primary care physician is the doctor with whom you build a relationship. Aside from perhaps an obstetrician/ gynecologist, this is the one instance where the personal relation-ship you have with the doctor is of the utmost importance. It's fine if the doctor who sets your broken leg or operates on your sinuses is personable and easy to talk to, but it's not essential to your care. But you need to have a primary care doctor with whom you can communicate. You need to feel comfortable talk-ing to your doctor about embarrassing physical ailments. You need to feel that you can trust your doctor. Without that core trust, your working relationship—and by extension, your med-ical care—is compromised.

The primary care doctor's role in your care is twofold. The doctor monitors your health over time, treats problems of a gen-eral nature, and builds up a bank of knowledge about your health habits and how you respond to basic treatments. If a problem arises that requires more specialized care, he or she provides referrals, serves as a filter for information, and keeps track as the situation evolves. The primary doctor is the voice of reason, the one that puts everything in context for you. In this sense, the internist acts something like command central, keeping tabs on where you are and what you need, interpreting all information as it relates to you, and delegating responsibility for different aspects of your care.

As with the choice of a medical center, your choice of a primary care physician affects every other subsequent choice in your medical care—even if it's not readily apparent. With your internist, you're getting a network of the physicians he or she knows and has worked with over many years. You're getting the collective wisdom of the physicians who have helped to train your doctor. You're getting a level of judgment and a philosophy that informs that judgment. You're getting service from the other doctors, nurses, and staff in your doctor's office. With so much riding on your choice of physician, you want that choice to be a good one.

But getting good care from your doctor is not a one-way issue. Your role in the patient-doctor relationship has an impact on your treatment as well. In this chapter, we'll take a look at how to locate a good primary care doctor and what *you* can do to ensure you get good care.

WHY YOU NEED A PRIMARY CARE DOCTOR

Many people say, "I'm healthy. Why do I need an internist? If a medical problem comes up, I can always go to see the appropriate subspecialist."

My answer to this is that beginning with a subspecialist is like starting your meal with dessert. You're not getting the benefit of a square meal. You think, "I have a gastrointestinal problem. I'll go right to the GI person and skip the internist." First of all, since you have diagnosed your own problem, you may not even be in the right place. But let's say you do find your way to the right specialist. He or she may be able to address your immediate problem, but won't have the benefit of ongoing knowledge about your health—knowledge that could aid your treatment. In this kind of situation, it's as though you're out on a raft in the middle of the sea. With a good specialist the raft may be quite sturdy, but you're not in continual contact with others as you should be.

Here's a simple illustration of how an internist demonstrates his value again and again. My husband was looking for a quality doctor to treat his sinuses. I could have called one of the ENT specialists I work with. The ENT could steer me toward a colleague who knows his stuff, but he wouldn't necessarily know how that colleague treats his patients. The internist, however, is accustomed to patients coming back after a referral and saying, "What a nice guy" or "I found him difficult to work with." Then, from a medical perspective, the internist will read the report and get an impression of the specialist's expertise and professionalism. With every referral, you're piggybacking on all the other referrals he or she has made.

The internist will make a judgment on several levels. One is patient satisfaction: the doctor's style, the ease of dealing with the doctor's office, how the system works. As a physician, the internist is saying, "Did the specialist solve the problem? Was I able to communicate with him?" So in that one referral my husband gets from his internist, there's a ten-point checklist behind it. There's no other effective way to get that.

If you have an ongoing relationship with an internist, he will have come to know your strengths and anxieties. Such a doctor is going to make a different referral than someone who doesn't know you. Let's say you need to see a specialist and your internist has two possibilities in mind. One guy is a toughie and the other is a softie. If you're an anxious sort, the toughie might not have time to sit and chat with you, whereas the softie might have a warmer, more relaxed style. Or, you may have a no-nonsense approach to your own health and be wary of someone with a touchy-feely manner. Either way, all this goes in the hopper as your internist makes a referral for you. If it's just a matter of getting a name, someone could arbitrarily pick one from a list. Either way, you're getting good care. But the care most fine-tuned for your needs can only come from someone who knows you.

People who don't have an internist often try to diagnose their own illnesses. This is not wise. You may think you know what's wrong with you, but not be exactly right. Being a little off can lead to disastrous decisions. You may decide on your own which doctor you think you should see only to go down the wrong road. You may not know what's wrong and be scared; rather than let fear drive your decisions, you need the clear head of an internist to sort things out. The fact is that if you know something's wrong and you have no clear diagnosis, you need a doctor to go to. Without a primary doctor running the show, everything tends to get muddled. No one is directing the flow of information. Ideally, you can tell your internist "this hurts" and your doctor says, "Let's take tests and get you to the right specialist."

A CAUTIONARY TALE

In the following case, the lack of an internist made things far messier than they needed to be.

An elderly woman was found to have uterine cancer. Her ob/gyn had been ignoring abnormal Pap smears over the course of several years. This wasn't malpractice; the results were borderline and thus a matter of judgment. I don't know if she knew about the Pap smears; maybe she didn't want to know. Anyway, she started to get abdominal pain. At this point, her daughter, a friend of mine, started orchestrating her care and setting up appointments with doctors. She took her to an oncologist who wanted to treat her with radiation and chemotherapy. A second oncologist suggested a slightly different regimen. A third concurred with the first. After going through a little chemotherapy, the woman said: "I'm not doing this." Several gynecological oncologists set up a conference to consult on her case and she didn't show up. Basically, she had checked herself out of the health care system.

A few months later she collapsed in her apartment. City law requires that when this happens, the patient must be taken to the nearest hospital. So she entered the hospital—unconscious, with a systemic infection (sepsis), bilateral pneumonia, and her kidneys

FINDING RELIABLE HEALTH INFORMATION

Among the primary care physician's many tasks is filtering out information for the patient. A tremendous amount of medical information is available to the general consumer today. However, you need information that's both credible and relevant to you. As a layperson, that can be hard to assess. Information on the internet is often wrong, uncensored, or extreme.

Medical organizations' websites can be the most useful. If you go to an online chat room for a particular medical problem, you might be overwhelmed by far more information than you ever wanted, or by patient reports that frighten you. The reason is that groups centered on a particular disease will address the entire spectrum of that disease. The people who spend time on chat rooms are often those who have unusual or extreme manifestations of a given condition— those most motivated to seek out fellow travelers. However, such content is hardly the kind that's going to ease your mind. More likely, you'll worry and confuse yourself unnecessarily.

The best way to get health information relevant to you is by channeling it through your physician. The doctor—or physician's assistant, or nurse, or office manager—can streamline the information for you and direct you to appropriate resources. This is one of your doctor's important functions, but not many patients take advantage of this service. Many consumers, in fact, take it upon themselves to become experts in any problem they think they might have. Given the fact that we can never know as much as someone with twenty years of experience seeing patients, it makes sense to turn to your doctor as a source of information.

shut down—without any primary care doctor to monitor the situation. She was on a respirator in the Intensive Care Unit (ICU) for four days. The hospital doctors took excellent care of her. Mind you, they were treating her without the benefit of previous information about her health. There was no supervising doctor for oncology or internal medicine. She was seeing all these different doctors, but there was no one to put things in perspective or deal with her overall care. This was not a matter of access or economics; this was a well-to-do, intelligent woman who had no problem affording the best care.

She left the hospital, still without a doctor. She had a metastatic disease and a mass in her abdomen that was affecting her bowel and other parts of her body. She did not feel well. Now what?

This woman was refusing treatment because she was afraid of the treatment. She had said, "I don't want treatment. I'm going to die." An internist's care would have been pivotal at this point. When she decided against treatment for the cancer—and it was her right to do so—an internist might have said, "Let's take a route somewhere in the middle and get you comfortable." An internist who knew her would have been her advocate with the subspecialist who didn't, and shouldn't have been expected to, know her. The internist could have dealt with her fear and said, "Let's figure out what works for you." Treatment often involves a negotiation. Everyone knows that patients may make different choices. It's never one-size-fits-all.

Because no one was there, foolish decisions were made. It was either "let's fix you" or "leave it alone." The specific problem— a theoretically treatable gynecological cancer—became a total body disease. The course of the disease may have been inevitable, but it didn't have to happen like this. If she wanted to die a peaceful death, this was not the way. And it certainly was not what she wanted.

If you don't have a primary care physician, start looking for one now. It's better to choose a physician when you're healthy

OB/GYNS AS PRIMARY CARE DOCTORS BY DEFAULT

Some women use their ob/gyn as their primary care doctor. Technically speaking, this is not okay. An ob/gyn will not have the broad network that a primary doctor does. Ob/gyns and other specialists are not qualified to do general internal medicine. They shouldn't, for example, be prescribing antibiotics for minor infections or in any way act as a substitute for an internist. However, many ob/gyns have accepted this role because they know that their patients need one practitioner that is a constant. Though not ideal, this is the accommodation many have made to serve their patients.

Many healthy young women understand the need to see a gynecologist on an annual basis but don't see the need to see an internist every year. If you're healthy, you probably don't need to go every year, but you do need at least to *have* an internist. Your doctor will tell you when you should check back. In selecting an internist, you're getting tapped into the medical network at another level. As ob/gyns don't interact with specialists in the same way, having one as your sole advocate skews your available referral network.

and thinking clearly than when disaster strikes and suddenly you need one. Maybe you're thinking, "I don't want to bother. I'm fine." The point is that, over time, all the exchanges and interactions you have with your doctor accumulate so that he or she knows you pretty well. If you confront an illness or emergency, this knowledge kicks in so that you get much better care than you would with a near-stranger running the show.

FINDING YOUR DOCTOR

A lawyer friend came to me with this question:

"My beloved internist of many years just retired. He suggested a younger internist. I went to the guy and I liked him. He recommended that I have a colonoscopy. How do I know that I really need this, and that he has no financial relationship with the doctor he was suggesting would do the procedure—you know, some kind of financial incentive?"

First I asked him which hospital the new internist was affiliated with, and determined that the doctors there were all good. After that, I told him that as a patient, you're stuck with honor and trust. There's no way around this. You can't possibly know every conceivable motivation for your doctor's recommendation, and you'll drive yourself crazy if you question everything he says. You need to trust your own instincts and decide: Is this doctor going to give me good care and good advice? A doctor you can trust is worth his weight in gold. But it's also up to you to give him that trust.

Then I turned the question around to him: If I came to him for legal advice and he suggested I see a more specialized lawyer, could I trust that his referral didn't involve some kind of payback? Frankly, he was insulted. I told him it was the exact same thing in medicine: There's a core of honor and expertise in the profession.

Since trust is a pretty big word, you want to take time to make your choice. As it is, many people spend less time picking their doctors than they would a pair of shoes. People select doctors for reasons like location, convenience, or "she seemed nice." People can tell you why they bought their car more easily than they can tell you why they chose their doctor. In my experience, people all too often don't take enough time to determine whom they go to, and then get angry at the results.

BEGINNING THE SEARCH

In the last chapter we discussed why choosing a medical institution is the best first step. Once you've narrowed the field by picking the hospital, you can take a multilevel approach to selecting a specific physician:

Get referrals from people you know. Everyone knows the scuttlebutt around town. Everyone has a co-worker, friend, or uncle who has seen a local doctor and has a story to tell. People are usually quite willing to share what they know, happily singing the praises of doctors they adore and complaining vociferously about those they don't like.

Ask the pros. If you know any health care workers on the hospital staff, ask which practices they prefer. Staff people know how doctors function in the hospital and how effective they are. They also know which doctors everyone respects.

Consult your insurance provider. Compare the list of affiliated doctors with your HMO or insurance list and see who matches up.

Call the American Board of Internal Medicine [(800) 441-ABIM]: Ask for doctors in your geographical area who are board-certified. You'll probably get the names of two or three doctors who are part of excellent groups.

Call the hospital. Most medical centers have a referral number, which can be helpful. But beyond this, hospital administrators can be a great resource. You can call the CEO's office at the hospital—don't worry, you're not going to get the CEO, you're going to get his or her administrative assistant—and say something like, "I'm a new patient and want to find a physician on your staff. Can you make a recommendation?" The administrator's orientation is to try to help the consumer. You won't necessarily get what you want, but you may get pretty close.

As you scout around, the same names will keep cropping up. Of these, choose two to interview. Learn their credentials so that you can be sure that they are competent, qualified, and who they represent themselves to be. Check with the American Board of _____ (pick whichever specialty applies), the highest credentialing body in the nation for each specialty. (For your con-
(continued on page 50.)

AND KEEP IN MIND...

If you're married...

It might be a good idea for both you and your husband to see the same group of doctors, though not necessarily the same doctor. They get to know you better, so you get better care. In the course of treating you, your doctor may need to talk to your spouse. For instance, if you get sick the doctor may want to give him or her instructions on caring for you at home. If one of you has a diagnosis, the doctor will deliver it to both of you. Knowing your partner enhances communication and makes your care better.

This is what my husband and I do. I go to one person in the group and my husband goes to another. I'm friends with the doctor he goes to. I don't want to be his patient. Quite frankly, I don't want to be buddies with my doctor or to have to undress in front of a friend. As my friend, he can't take care of me properly.

You may wonder if having doctors in the same group is a little too cozy. Let's say there's a delicate matter. A man says, "I don't want my wife to know I have a venereal disease." In the medical field, confidentiality trumps everything else. If you want to discuss something personal with your doctor, be assured that no one else will know. If you still have any reservations you can specifically say, "I want you to understand that this is strictly between us," so as to remind the doctor. The doctor can then make a confidential record.

If you do a significant amount of traveling...

As a frequent flyer, you might look for a physician who has a lot of international connections. In any event, you will want to tell your physician that you do travel. Depending on your illness (e.g., diabetes, cardiac, arthritis, high blood pressure) your doctor will give you a copy of your medical records and relevant lab tests, such as an EKG. Similarly, he or she can give you a complete medical summary which includes important tests.

Find out about your doctor's international connections. Doctors vary greatly as to how tapped in they are. Recently I helped a newborn baby in Dubai who had meningitis. I have found doctors in Hong Kong, London, and Switzerland. In general, people at nationally ranked medical centers are more likely to function on an international level.

If you have an ongoing medical problem...

Say you're dealing with an ongoing medical problem like arthritis, irritable bowel disease, diabetes, a heart-related illness, or a significant family medical history. You might choose a general internist who has expertise in that area. This way you're not constantly running off to a subspecialist. Also, when you do consult your subspecialist, the internist is well equipped to interpret and explain. A physician may have completed a fellowship in cardiology and have chosen to practice internal medicine rather than be a practicing cardiologist full time. It's a little like one-stop shopping. Having an internist trained in cardiology doesn't mean that you don't go to the cardiologist. This merely tailors your care more specifically to you.

You can ask about the different areas of expertise within the group. Some groups have several specialties represented, something like a department store with cardiology, endocrinology, rheumatology, gastroenterology, etc.

If location is one of your main concerns...

You might be worrying about how the doctor's location will fit in with your schedule. You may, for example, want to have a doctor who's closest to your workplace rather than your home. However, given that—with the possible exception of pediatricians—you're not likely to be visiting your primary care doctor on a regular basis, it's worth trading off your inconvenience for the physician's expertise.

(continued from page 47.)
venience, a listing of the specialty boards can be found on page X.) At that point, you can set up interviews to see which one of the two you bond with, or what works the best for you.

INTERVIEWING YOUR DOCTOR

Most insurance companies don't reimburse for interviews per se. If you can find some way to afford it, don't let cost stand in your way. It's a good investment. Otherwise, go for a first exam. As long as there is a "diagnosis," you will be reimbursed.

Pediatricians are used to being interviewed by prospective parents. Internists, however, are not accustomed to this. But you needn't fear that you are in any way wasting your money (you're not) or wasting their time. A primary care physician wants to know how you fit him as well as how he fits you.

Basically, what you get from the interview is a sense of the person. To a large extent, the answers you're getting are not direct responses to your questions. Rather, you're gathering impressions about this person from body language and personal manner.

If you have specific concerns, you can ask about competence in that area. If you're healthy, you can ask about the doctor's philosophy of practice. Every physician has one. Let's say the doctor describes himself as a big believer in preventive medicine. Does this mean that he or she suggests vitamins or encourages routine screening tests? Find out.

Ask about the doctor's approach to medical care. Pose the question, "If I need to see a subspecialist, will you follow me through the process, interpreting test results and counseling me? Or am I on my own?"

Many people think they don't know enough to question their doctor. But you needn't be an M.D. yourself to engage in a discussion about your medical care. It's like shopping for a car: Even if you don't know how the engine works, at least you will know if the relative quality compares to similar cars.

Don't worry about the conversation. With a good doctor, it will take care of itself. Doctors know that everyone brings something to the appointment. For example, someone may say, "My father died of a heart attack at age fifty and I'm about to turn fifty myself." A good doctor will pick up on this. Doctors actively look for the indirect message. This is a skill we've been taught.

You will certainly respond in a visceral way to the doctor's manner and personality. But remember that a medical appointment demands a different etiquette than ordinary social interactions. For example, don't be put off if, during your conversation, the doctor interrupts you. The physician needs to keep tight control over the pace of the session. First, it is a rare physician who has enough time to let a conversation meander. But also, it is a rare patient who knows how to offer a good medical history. The doctor may lead with questions and may steer the discussion in a certain direction. Sometimes the doctor may do this too quickly, in which case you might feel rushed. If you left something out, tell him later in the exam or, if you're already home, call and leave a message with the receptionist that the doctor should call you back.

This is why every doctor's office will have you fill out those lengthy checklists. The doctor needs to organize information about your medical condition in a certain way. The information from the form combined with what you relate will give the doctor a foundation from which to direct your care.

Despite all this advance preparation, you won't know how your doctor is going to be in different situations. As with most things in life, you find out the hard way as you go along. However, there are certain things you can find out ahead of time:

- ✓ How long has the physician been in practice?
- ✓ Is the physician a board-certified internist? Or, if a family practitioner, certified by the American Board of Family Practice? Determine the physician's level of training so that you understand his or her place in the

pecking order. The physician should formally explain his or her credentials in language you can understand.

✓ Is the office clean or dirty?

✓ Is the staff courteous?

✓ Are the office hours convenient for you? (Some offices have evening and weekend hours; others don't. If you're tethered to your desk from nine to five, this may make a difference to you.)

✓ Is the doctor on your plan?

✓ How do they bill? Some offices will fill out the insurance forms and send them in. Some have you do it, and still others bill you immediately for the differential.

✓ How do they handle emergencies? If you get sick and need to go to the hospital, where do they send you?

✓ How do they facilitate communication? Is there a specified time during which patients can call the doctor? You can ask the doctor: "If I have a significant question, how do I get to you?" Each office has a chain of command for information. As a patient, it's your job to find it out. The message you want to give your doctor is, "I'll do it your way. What is your way?" Some doctors use email now. I often call patients back after my son goes to bed. For me it's easier to have a conversation without ringing phones and other distractions. I let patients know that this is my plan. I don't want people sitting by the phone waiting. When you're nervous and sick, your anxiety over not getting an answer goes up. You need to have confidence that you're being cared for. If they don't respond in a timely way to your polite requests for information—on their schedule—then your doctor isn't taking care of you.

✓ Will you always be seeing your doctor, or might you be seeing others in the practice?

WORKING WITH YOUR INSURANCE

Don't assume that an expensive insurance plan will automatically land you a top-tier doctor. Similarly, less than premium coverage doesn't necessarily preclude your getting the best doctors. Low level insurance plans can provide super doctors or reimburse you for seeing one when a given specialty isn't on their roster. You still must check the doctor's credentials, but if you have a lower level of coverage, you may have to work harder to get the credentials of the physicians within the system. The insurance company may not make this information immediately accessible to you. You may need someone to translate the insurance company's list of doctors to determine the doctor's affiliation and credentials.

Here is a strategy to use: Use the hospital or medical center as a starting point. Find the appropriate department within the hospital and ask which doctors are on your particular insurance company's list. If you have already checked out the medical center, you know all the physicians there are of a certain caliber. On any given list of doctors, some are better, some are good, and some are merely okay. It's worth making the effort to get the physician affiliated with the superior hospital.

WHEN IT'S SMART TO GO
OUTSIDE YOUR INSURANCE

You aren't absolutely locked into your insurance list. There are "out of network" reimbursements at a lower rate. Or you can choose to go off the grid and pay directly for service. There are times when it's worth the investment.

A smart strategy: Go to the physicians on your insurance list for general care. Then, if you get a diagnosis, you can consider sidestepping the list in order to get a second opinion from someone truly excellent.

For example, a business associate of my husband's had a breast cancer scare. She found a lump and needed a biopsy. She called me to decode her insurance company's list of doctors.

There weren't any breast cancer specialists in any New York hospital on the list. Then we looked at medical centers, and we picked the best general surgeon at the best hospital.

I told her to go with the doctor on her insurance list for the initial step, the biopsy. She would also get the invisible doctors at the medical center: the anesthesiologist, radiologist, and, if needed, the pathologist. If there was a problem, the pathologist was going to determine her fate in a case like this, and he came along with the doctor. Then, if anything showed up and it looked as if the case would involve some higher-order judgment, she could go off-list and consult with a breast cancer specialist. As it turned out, the biopsy was negative so she didn't need to go further. But this way she covered her bases. She took the first step without having to spend a lot of money and held the top specialist in reserve should the situation take a more complicated turn.

Note that not all physicians accept insurance. Some have stopped taking it because of difficulties getting reimbursed; unfortunately, this is becoming more prevalent. Such doctors charge on a fee-for-service basis.

CHANGING PRIMARY CARE DOCTORS

You might consider switching doctors for two reasons: One, if you feel that you and your doctor aren't a good "match"; and two, if the doctor has been negligent in your care. In the latter case, the sooner the better.

Several years ago, my husband was having elective back surgery, which required a complete preoperative examination including a chest X-ray and blood work. The internist was supposed to give the surgeon a letter with my husband's complete medical history. This included all of his previous surgery, any current diseases or medications, his weight, blood pressure, and the results of his latest physical examination. This was all necessary data for the anesthesiologist.

I told my husband to check with his doctor's office to see what had been sent. He got his doctor on the phone and asked about the blood work. The doctor said, "Don't worry about it. I didn't do any blood tests." My husband remembered quite vividly—this isn't the kind of thing you forget—that blood had been drawn. The doctor (1) had no record of this; (2) denied that the blood test had even occurred; and (3) didn't seem to think this was a matter of concern. They had to draw more blood for a repeat series of blood tests. While no fun, this wasn't a terribly big deal. But many tests are expensive, complicated, or uncomfortable, in which case repeating one *would* be a problem.

Most troubling to me, however, was that the doctor clearly had no intention of following up on the blood work to see if it had been done and what it revealed. And he had *no* intention of writing the requested report. The doctor wasn't being thorough, and thoroughness is the hallmark of a good primary care doctor. (Medical students are taught that it's the day-to-day, lab-test-to-lab-test detective work, leaving no stone unturned, making no assumptions, that makes the best physcians. No amount of academic scientific integrity can supplant the dogged legwork of checking lab tests and running down X-ray results. To be a good doctor, you don't have to be a genius, just compulsive.)

I urged my husband to get a new internist. He was upset because he liked his doctor and had seen him for a number of years. He protested that he was comfortable with his internist, who had a reputation for being very intelligent. But I prevailed. In my mind, there was no question about it. If this doctor had bungled something this simple, what would he do when it became complicated? I didn't want to find out at the expense of my husband's health.

At one point, I wondered whether I myself needed a new sub-specialist. I was anxious about this; I was dissatisfied with the care I was receiving but wasn't sure whether I was being reasonable.

I discussed this with my primary care doctor, who told me to make the appointment with the new person and see how I liked him. At that point, I could sever the link with the previous doctor. However, I should definitely not cut ties before deciding that I liked the new doctor. Of course, I thought. That makes perfect sense. The point is that everyone, even professionals, are cowed by this. The new subspecialist was, in fact, quite wonderful. In retrospect, I wondered why I hesitated.

Although it can be difficult for the average patient to judge a doctor on his or her expertise, keep in mind that temperament is a valid factor for consideration. A doctor can be nice or a grouch and none of it affects quality. If you're not happy with a doctor's style, it's not that they're not good, it's that they're not good for you. And that's reason enough to explore other options. It turned out that one doctor was better for me than the other. The first one wasn't a bad doctor. She just wasn't the best one for me.

So if you're not happy with your physicians, try out the new one first. You want to be sure that the grass is greener. If you decide to make the switch, request that your records be sent to you. Some doctors don't like to release records, but this is their obligation and your legal right. Then get the records to the new doctor. It's also not a bad idea to keep a copy of your records, especially if you have conditions that require monitoring.

BE PROACTIVE WITH YOUR GENERAL MEDICAL CARE

To get the most out of your primary care doctor, you need to take charge of your medical care. Here are some tips to help you become a responsible and informed patient:

Make a mini-medical record to keep with you at all times. Type up a list of the medications you're taking on a credit card-sized paper and keep this in your wallet. Or, you can shrink the information from a regular 8½-by-11-inch piece of paper. The reason: When you're hurt or nervous, you can't think straight. A doctor treating you in an emergency needs to know what you take and whether it's 25 mg or 50 mg or some other dose. Some drugs might have adverse reactions with other drugs, or could affect test results. (Note: If you're a cardiac patient, you should also have your latest EKG reduced to card size somewhere on your person.)

Keep your doctor informed. If you're out of the country and have an emergency, the first thing to do is call your own primary care doctor because he or she can assess the current problem within the context of your overall health. Your doctor (or your doctor's associate) can then get on the phone with the doctor who's treating you and discuss the situation. The office will have your chart and a list of your medications, which can then be faxed to the doctor abroad. (Ideally, if you travel a great deal, you should have with you a full report from your primary care doctor, with medications, EKGs, and the most recent lab results.) As things evolve, your doctor can run interference for you and tell you which hospital in the area to go to. The telephone is a wonderful thing. Use it.

Find out how your doctor's office handles spur-of-the-moment situations. With emergencies, some practices will have you call the office and go to the emergency room. Others prefer for general "I need an answer today" questions that you call first thing in the morning, and they'll make sure that you get seen that day. If all you need is to talk with your doctor, see if you can establish a brief time for you to call the doctor or be available at that time so that the doctor can call you. Someone from the office should be available all the time. Sunday at 1:00 A.M. is just another hour in the medical business. Someone will be on call, and your records are always available.

Don't be afraid to call your doctor between appointments to ask a question. Many people have questions but worry that they're not worth bothering the doctor about. The truth is that very rarely do people call me with unnecessary questions. The ones who do so tend to do it repeatedly. This quickly becomes known to the office staff, who then sort through the questions first. The vast majority of the time, I find that behind every "stupid" question is a valid medical concern.

There is an etiquette to dealing with medical professionals. But if you're mindful of that, you're unlikely to transgress, much the way that you're unlikely to barge into your neighbor's home and sit down in the middle of their dinner. If something is worrying you, call your doctor. That's what your doctor is there for.

THE WELL-CHOREOGRAPHED WELL-VISIT

You think that a basic medical exam is something that the doctor does to you. But guess what: you're doing it together. In any exam, your doctor is examining you *with* you. It's not a matter of you lying quietly on the examining table until the doctor announces, "I found the problem." The more you participate, the more effective the exam and the better for you.

At the opening of an annual physical, the doctor will ask you questions or engage you in what seems to be idle chit-chat. The doctor is trying to make you comfortable and find out how you're doing. In asking, "What's happened since I last saw you?" he's finding out which specialists you've seen in the intervening time. When the doctor asks, "How's your sex life?" he wants to know that you're physiologically sound; certain diseases cause orgasmic and erection difficulty. Every question is part of the doctor's detective work. All these details about your health are related. A fragment of information here, a fragment there, and the doctor starts putting the pieces together.

The exam itself is so brief that you don't want any wasted time. As a patient, you have to map out what you're going to say. Essentially, it's like Hollywood, where you've got five minutes to make a pitch for a movie script. Keep in mind that this isn't because the doctor wants it this way. Quite simply, this is the reality we are all living in. The doctor is aware that he needs to direct traffic. Doctors know that patients do not speak the language of physicians and that they may need to ferret out the information they need.

A standard office visit runs less than fifteen minutes, even less than ten minutes in our new world of medical care. There's a bit of a dance as the two of you balance what the patient wants from the doctor with what the doctor wants from the patient. The doctor will develop a line of questions in response to any articulated concerns. Over time, as trust and familiarity between patient and doctor build, this process becomes more efficient and complete.

As a patient, you can make the appointment work for you. Here's how:

Write your questions down in advance. Many people—myself included—forget their name the minute they walk into a doctor's office. If you're prone to forget things on the spot, write down questions. Don't worry about having too many; often several questions may relate to the same problem. The list of questions will keep you on track so that you don't walk out and think, "Oh no, I forgot to ask about...." You can simply hand the list to the doctor as you go in, and he'll work the questions into the exam.

When you're writing the list, start at the top of the body and work your way down. This way, when you get to an embarrassing subject you don't have to say anything. Rather, your doctor can say, "I see you're concerned about an itch," and all you have to do is say, "Yeah, I have an itch." Everyone knows certain ailments are awkward to talk about. The point is you want to make it easy for your doctor to take care of you.

Keep an open mind. Don't go into the visit convinced that you know what is wrong with you and what should be done. Everyone's always diagnosing their own problems—incorrectly, I might add. Having a primary care doctor who knows you and has cared for you over time takes this burden off you.

Be open to the possibility that nothing needs to be done. People think that if they go into a doctor's appointment with a complaint and don't come back with a diagnosis or a prescription, they've wasted their time. This isn't so. Actually, the most difficult thing for a doctor is to say nothing's wrong. There are always little odds and ends that aren't quite right. The doctor has to make a judgment as to whether this is part of a disease process.

Tell the doctor everything you're taking. Every over-the-counter medication or herbal preparation has medical implications, so make sure your doctor knows about them. Don't think, "It's just an aspirin" so you needn't mention it. An aspirin is an anticoagulant, and taking aspirin regularly can affect the course of surgery.

I once operated on a paramedic who had been seen by twenty doctors in five operations in the aftermath of a car accident. I was fixing his eye, and saw that he was oozing more than normal. The anesthesiologist mentioned that he had a coagulation deficiency (a blood-clotting problem). The paramedic had told neither me nor his neurosurgeon, even upon direct questioning! Before I did a second operation, he had received coagulation factors from a hematologist, who then cleared him for surgery. This suggests the kind of risk presented by a lack of coagulation factors, which is similar to what taking aspirin can do.

Don't belittle your concerns. The dynamic of doctor appointments is such that, typically, the patient feels embarrassed and the doctor is busy. This is true even when the patient is a doctor. The problem doesn't have to be specifically "medical." If you're in pain because your world is falling down around you, that's not okay. If you have chronic headaches that you attribute to stress, that's not okay. Don't dismiss your problems by saying, "Well, I'm not dying tomorrow." Your doctor's job is to help you and you're entitled to ask for help.

Be honest about your level of compliance. We're all cagey about these things. The doctor tells you to do X, Y, and Z, and you only do X and Y.

When I lecture to third year medical students, I describe the difficulty presented by a form of amblyopia (a significant loss of vision in one eye) treatment in which a patch is put over the seeing eye, forcing the child to use the poorer seeing eye in an attempt to strengthen it. When I talk about how hard this is to impose, I often get glazed looks. But when I ask if anyone has ever cheated on a diet or if they universally take all their antibiotics four times daily for seven days, everyone gives a knowing, if uncomfortable, laugh.

If you're honest, the doctor can better understand why a given treatment didn't work. For example, if you still have an infection, it's helpful for the doctor to know whether or not you took the entire course of antibiotics. It's not that you're a good patient or bad patient. It's that you're the patient and your doctor needs the facts in order to treat you.

Don't save the best for last. I can't tell you how often I'm halfway out the door after what I thought was a complete examination when the patient raises a topic of great concern. Do not wait until the end of an appointment to mention chest pain, blood in your stool, numbness throughout your arm, erectile dysfunction, vaginal discharge, or an occasional loss of vision in one eye.

This may sound obvious, but people often downplay the importance of such symptoms or spend the bulk of the session building up enough courage to mention them. You want your doctor to be able to use your appointment time wisely, so it's important to mention matters of importance right up front.

A good time to mention something personal is when the doctor's back is turned—literally. It's the same principle as the

Catholic confessional or Freud's couch: People are more candid when the listener isn't looking straight at them.

Another reason to describe unusual symptoms first is that your doctor may vary his physical examination depending on what's bothering you. For example, conditions like diabetes and gastrointestinal problems involve areas of your body you wouldn't think of. If you've already gotten dressed, you'll have to undress again and start the entire process over.

Call with questions. A fine physician will end the examination by asking if the patient has any questions remaining or if there's anything else you want him or her to be aware of. Use this opportunity well. But the door needn't be closed once you leave. If, as often happens, questions occur to you on your way home, put in a call to the office.

Dealing with parents, I know that questions might not arise until after the children have gone to bed and the parents have time to talk and think things over. During the examination, they may have been attending to or worrying about the child. I make it clear to the parents that I will be available to them later. Their concerns are not a now-or-never issue.

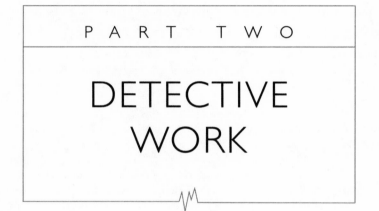

PART TWO

DETECTIVE WORK

MUCH OF MEDICINE INVOLVES detective work. In order to help a patient, a physician needs to know (1) exactly what the patient is suffering from; and (2) what to do about it. As often as not, the answers to these questions are not obvious. Not all illnesses follow the textbook version with all of the classic signs and symptoms. Similarly, the treatment picture is rarely clear and predictable. The physician serving as the "detective" on the case will assemble relevant clues, some straightforward and some subtle, and put together working hypotheses for both the diagnosis and the recommended course of action.

The challenge of determining a diagnosis and recommending treatment amidst uncertainty makes this work interesting and rewarding to the doctor. Not that you should care about your doctor's level of intellectual engagement—and certainly no patient wants to be the fascinating case discussed around the lunch table—but this gives you a glimpse of what your doctor is up to. This is the art of medicine. It draws on science but also involves the intangibles: instinct, intuition, and experience.

As a patient, you can do your part to minimize the guesswork by (1) making sure that you're consulting the right medical specialist(s); and (2) ensuring that any specialists are given all needed information. Also, understanding the process of pinpointing diagnoses and treatments will help you appreciate exactly what your physician is doing for you, keep your expectations realistic, and clarify your role throughout. In addition, the more you know about how this works in practice, the more vigilant you can be.

Over the next three chapters, we discuss what you need to know about the various components of medical sleuthing: coming up with a diagnoses; choosing an appropriate treatment; and making the best use of second opinions.

CHAPTER FOUR

Diagnosis

P UT SIMPLY, A DIAGNOSIS IS what's wrong with you. When you know that something is wrong, but you don't know what, you need to get a diagnosis. The diagnosis is a prerequisite to deciding upon a course of treatment.

In making the diagnosis, the doctor wants to be able to narrow it down as specifically as possible. The diagnosis needs to be precise, for it will determine everything that follows. As the doctor examines you, he or she is mentally running through a line of questions, the answers to which will begin to situate your problem. The doctor is thinking: What category of problem are we dealing with? Where is it located—the head, the chest, the digestive tract?

You can divide diseases into two basic groups. In one group, regional diseases, the problem is exactly where it looks like it is. You have an ear infection; you have pain in your ear. The other group of diseases are systemic; they affect many parts of the body. Ulcerative colitis, a disease of the digestive tract, can cause problems in the eyes. Lyme disease can cause headaches, joint pain, and digestive troubles. Many diseases are global, but as a patient, you're not thinking globally. You're thinking, "It hurts where it hurts." A patient may wonder, "Why is the guy looking in my eyes when it's my knees that ache?" The reason probably is that he suspects arthritis. With arthritis, you get a specific type of inflammatory reaction in the front of your eye. It is painless and doesn't always affect vision, so you won't necessarily know that you have it. This is what the doctor is looking for. Finding disease in a secondary site can help establish a diagnosis, as well as suggest the progression and severity of the illness.

The point for the patient is this: You can't always understand the detective thought processes. It's like Detective Friday on *Dragnet*, or any other famous private eye. What goes through the doctor's mind is not what's going on in your mind. You each have entirely different tapes running through your head. A good diagnostician is busily putting the pieces together while you're still in the dark.

A diagnostic sixth sense is a gift. A doctor with this particular gift is always ten mental steps ahead of everyone else. The trick to diagnosis is figuring out where to look. It's a lot like the art of dowsing, figuring out where water lies under the ground. A true diagnostician intuitively knows where to look, picking up on tiny clues that slide beneath others' awareness. This is the person who puts together a dinosaur from a single bone in the toe, while others would need half of the skeleton to do so. In a given hospital, everyone knows who the top diagnosticians are, among both generalists and specialists. People will know who can best answer a particular question. If you start with an internist who's a crack diagnostician, you're already ahead of the game.

Today, doctors are trained to rely on tools for diagnosis as well as observational skills. We're more dependent on tests and X-rays because we have so much technology available to us. Quite simply, we're spoiled. If you go to another country, even England or Canada, you'll see that doctors have fewer technological diagnostic tools and therefore use them less. And in the United States, the really good people will still see the whole diagnostic picture and rely on observation and judgment as well as on what the tests say.

Ultimately, the diagnosis will be based on a compilation of many puzzle pieces, many of which are tangible (based on observation and tests) and others that are intangible (based on judgment). A great deal of knowledge and experience goes into interpreting the various signs (e.g., a swollen knee) and symptoms (e.g., "my knee hurts"). As a patient, you want to be sure that the information that goes into the diagnosis file is accurate *and* that it goes to the right person—the physician best qualified to draw conclusions from it. That's why you want to be sure that you're working with doctors, generalists as well as specialists, with the highest level of certification. Doctors with board-certification (the American Board of X specialty), have demonstrated knowledge—and the use of that knowledge. All diagnosticians are not equal. By seeking doctors of a known quality, you're increasing your luck. Because in the end, you're essentially left with your physician's judgment.

While your doctor is hunting down the diagnosis, you might feel as if you should stay out of the way. However, your instincts are important, and you must make sure to articulate them. A friend of mine, Linda, had a family history of breast cancer. When she felt a lump in her breast, she went to see her doctor immediately. Her doctor, however, did not feel a mass, and the mammogram was normal. Nevertheless, Linda was concerned. She stood her ground and said, "I have a lump, and I would like it checked out." Respecting her instincts and her wishes, the physician suggested an ultrasound, which showed that there was indeed a lump. When the lump was biopsied, it was found to be cancerous. Today, Linda has gone through bilateral mastectomies and reconstructive surgery, but she's alive. She had a feeling that something was wrong—that it needed to be checked out—and she made sure that it was. This was the right thing to do.

ZEROING IN ON THE PROBLEM

In determining your diagnosis, your doctor is making a precise evaluation of what you have. He or she is measuring your symptoms against those that typify a particular disease, going back and forth between your presentation and what is known about an illness until finding an exact fit. The precision is important because there are so many variations of each disease. For instance, all cases of pneumonia are not the same. A diagnosis of pneumonia would mean one thing in a healthy person without a preexisting cold, another in someone with a tumor when the lung area has shown up cloudy on an X-ray, and yet another in an elderly person when the pneumonia is a secondary infection. Each case would be treated a different way.

To illustrate a doctor's thinking at the diagnosis stage, let's look at the disease diabetes, which can produce a broad range of problems. Diabetes is an elevated level of blood glucose (sugar) often due to insulin resistance. You may also get problems with blood vessels in the eyes; this would be determined by an eye exam. Or you could have kidney problems; this would be detected via specialized blood and urine tests. Or you could have impeded blood flow to the extremities, possibly leading to ulcers in the feet or legs or altered sensation in your feet or hands.

A doctor could say, "You have diabetes. Let's look for the five most common manifestations of the disease to get a clearer picture of the illness." Or, the doctor might think, "I'm seeing someone with a leg ulcer. This leads me to ask: Does this patient have diabetes?" In other words, it works both ways. The doctor can work the diagnosis from the disease to the manifestations of that illness, or from the presentation to the disease. The doctor can enter the diagnostic process at different points. It all depends on how the patient presents his or her case.

So when you talk to a doctor about a problem like a leg ulcer, the ulcer itself could be the problem or it could be but one representation of an entire bouquet of problems. But to you, your immediate concern is that your leg hurts.

Take a common ailment, the headache. A headache could result from a simple problem like tension or allergies. Or it could relate to a more serious but still fairly common problem like a sinus infection, a vision problem, or a systemic inflammation as seen in Lyme disease. It could also be a migraine. Or, most rarely and seriously, an aneurysm or brain tumor. The pattern will tend to be specific to one type of headache. That's what the diagnostician will be looking for. But they may overlap. This is why the diagnostician will continually run through a mental checklist of the various headache types.

If the headache seems to follow a pattern that suggests tension—maybe it's worse on days you work with a particular boss—and it's relieved by common pain medication like aspirin, ibuprofen, or acetaminophen, you're set. But if the pain medication doesn't touch it and it's the worst headache you've ever had and the doctor knows you (this is where an ongoing relationship with your primary doctor comes in), your doctor may start to suspect something serious.

In working toward a diagnosis, a doctor has to consider all the facts in the context of your life. In today's medical system, more and more doctors who don't know their patients are being forced to make these judgments. If I call my doctor and say, "Something is definitely wrong. I'm having the worst headache of my life without anything else going on to explain it," after a few more questions my doctor may well suggest that I immediately get a CT scan. If I do have an aneurysm, the speed at which we act can be crucial. If, on the other hand, I don't have my own doctor, I would no doubt eventually make my way to the local emergency room, go through the process, and see a doctor who doesn't know me. But several critical hours may have gone by.

Most people with headaches don't have aneurysms, of course. But the point is that to the untrained observer, in the beginning all headaches frequently look the same. The winnowing-down process is a bit like what you go through when you're buying a car. At the most general level, all cars look the same. They all have four wheels, metal doors, a top, and a bottom. That's not specific enough. If you're looking for a metallic blue, eight-air-bag, seven-passenger, three-row, midsized, four-wheel-drive model, there's only one that matches exactly. A diagnosis has to approximate that level of precision.

The best approach in most circumstances is to use a working hypothesis. The doctor says, "I think the problem is X. Now, let's prove it." People often think that the diagnosis just pops out of you. But it's not that way at all. Often it takes several steps and several different viewpoints. Everyone wants this process to be straightforward. It's not. This makes it very interesting for us, and very frustrating for the patient.

TESTS FOR DIAGNOSIS

How do you get your diagnosis? You go to your internist and say, "The pain is here (specify place) in my body," and the doctor goes to work with his internal checklist, filing away some possible causes and eliminating others. Then the doctor may order some preliminary tests. These would include blood and urine tests or X-rays or both. In the case of lumps and bumps, a biopsy may be recommended. Double-check (1) that the results get to the doctor, and (2) that they are accurate.

How do you do this? Keep a list of all X-rays taken and other important tests, with the dates. Within a reasonable period of time—a few days or a week, depending on the test—make certain that your doctor has reviewed them, and that you know what the results are. All tests generate information that provides the basis for a diagnosis. If the tests are inaccurate or the results are ignored, the doctor's conclusions and subsequent treatment will be wrong.

A college professor friend of mine, Margaret, had just had outpatient stomach surgery and started to feel ill. The surgery was on a Tuesday and on Thursday she called the covering surgeon (her surgeon was away). "You are fine," she was told. Over the weekend, she took herself to the local emergency room, as she was having trouble breathing. They took X-rays and sent her home. The next week she went back to her surgeon, who called and checked on the X-rays and found that they had revealed double pneumonia. The ER doctor had not even checked them! Her surgeon was enraged; her pneumonia had been left untreated for a week. Here she was, not a young woman, already weakened by the surgery, and all she needed was an antibiotic to treat the pneumonia. The ER had done the right thing by taking the X-ray, but the best tests are useless if nobody looks at them.

Margaret had fallen through the cracks. Knowing that this happens sometimes, what could she have done differently? She could have insisted on seeing the covering surgeon. Or, she could have called her primary care physician. As things were, she was adrift on her own. Even so, she could have refused to leave the emergency room until she had the results of the test. Before walking out of the emergency room, a patient can, and should, insist on having complete information from the visit.

If your diagnosis involves a biopsy of a tumor, the pathologist will play a key role in determining your situation. The word tumor simply means a growth. It could be a cancerous (malignant) growth, or it could be noncancerous (benign). Even if it's benign, it may cause discomfort or interfere with other organs. Though the very thought of a tumor is scary, the number of benign tumors greatly exceeds the number of cancerous tumors. As with other medical practitioners, pathologists have their own areas of expertise, such as breast tumors or polyps from the colon.

Make sure that you, the patient, know what has been removed or biopsied. You can't necessarily depend on anyone else to do the appropriate follow-up.

You're entitled to a written pathology report, along with the specific diagnosis. You need to understand what you have. Even if the tumor or cyst is benign, there may be variations that have different implications. Some benign lesions have a precancerous pattern. These results would be in the gray zone—not normal, but not cancerous. You need to know if your condition should be followed in the future, by whom, and how often. Every single time someone takes a piece out of you, you need to know what that piece revealed.

You want good people reading your tests. As with everything else in medicine, you make sure to get good people by choosing a good institution. Recently, my Uncle Herbie had a result on his PSA (Prostate Specific Antigens) test that warranted a biopsy to be sure he didn't have prostate cancer. His internist had sent him to a local urologist at the hospital he was affiliated with for a biopsy. He liked his local internist and wanted to stay with him. I tried to persuade him to have the test through Columbia-Presbyterian, noting that their pathology department is superior and that it's the pathologist, not his urologist or internist, who's the key player here. Reluctant to switch, he said, "Why don't I get the initial biopsy at my hospital? Then, if they find anything and need another biopsy, I can have the Columbia laboratory do it."

On the surface that seemed a logical compromise. But medicine doesn't work that way. I explained: "Once you do a biopsy, the area around the sample will have more scarring. Then you're dealing with something more complicated, which will make it harder to get a clean biopsy." The smart approach is to start with the top lab to get the clearest readings and the cleanest samples from the outset. "Now will you go to my hospital?" I asked him.

FINE-TUNING THE DIAGNOSIS

Your internist may also send you to an appropriate subspecialist to fine-tune the diagnostic picture. For unexplained headaches, you might go to a neurologist. For diabetes, an endocrinologist.

For sinuses, an ear, nose, and throat specialist (ENT). The key is that your internist is dispatching you to a specialist who will help define the problem *in conjunction with* him or her. Your internist will collaborate on your treatment with the specialist, or the internist will send you to the specialist for your treatment and remain in contact with both of you.

Ongoing communication between the internist and the specialist is important. Each has valuable information that the other needs. When a physician sends a patient to me for an evaluation, I always write to the referring doctor afterward. This is for (1) better patient care; (2) a copy of my exam for his records; (3) etiquette. I may say, "I didn't find a specific problem in my area of expertise, but there is a problem in someone else's camp." The primary care doctor can then contact a specialist in the next most likely area.

Let's say I am asked to examine a child who has headaches. I rule out eyestrain and eye muscle problems, myopia or the need for glasses, and other eye-based diseases. I fail to find any subtleties of headaches that pertain to my specialization. But the child still has the headaches. I may then suggest that the pediatrician send the child to a pediatric neurologist. After I've seen the child, the pediatrician can cross several possible diagnoses off the list and begin to think within a new paradigm. This is how the specialist and the primary care doctor work together.

The process is a lot like the game of Clue, with the doctor coming up with possible hypotheses and routing the patient to the proper subspecialist for that scenario. When the patient or the patient's family try to devise the route themselves, they make mistakes, at a cost of much money and discomfort. Each specialist sees a patient from his or her perspective, like overlapping floodlights. It's extremely difficult for a patient to choose the appropriate specialist.

The job of the specialist is to reread the tea leaves from his unique perspective. He or she may well see different shapes and patterns than the primary care doctor. If you go to someone with a bigger diagnostic vocabulary, there is a greater possibility of what you can find. This is true *even* if you do the same tests.

The more you can take advantage of your doctor's expertise, the better. If your doctor recommends that you see a certain specialist, you may not know every factor that went into that recommendation. For example, if a child needs a basic pair of glasses, a pediatrician is unlikely to send the child to me. If the situation seems more complex, I'll get the referral.

The other role your internist plays is that of translator. When a specialist is fine-tuning a diagnosis, he's speaking in a different language. It can get quite esoteric. Even the tools used to secure the diagnosis—fancy X-rays like MRIs and CT scans, subtle blood or genetic tests—can leave you feeling as if your were floating in a bowl of alphabet soup. You need to have your diagnosis explained to you clearly. Most often, the internist does this in conjunction with the specialist. If you speak to the specialist, make sure he or she speaks to you in terms that you understand. You can ask the specialist: "When you saw something like this before, what happened?" or "Among ten people who had this, what happened?"

MISTAKES YOU CAN NIP IN THE BUD

As a patient, you need somebody to keep a diary of your case. Document specifics like, "A test was done on such-a-such a date." Make sure that each test has been read and that you know the results. If there are any discrepancies, call your doctor's attention to them. If the results look bizarre, check into it. Perhaps left and right were flipped, or your tests were switched with someone else's. Such instances are rare, but they do happen. (See Chapter Eleven, The Patient's Advocate.)

A MATTER OF LEFT AND RIGHT

A third-year medical student I know told me about a faulty diagnosis in his own care that, had he not caught it, would have led to an unnecessary—and uncomfortable—procedure.

Jonas's dermatologist had been following moles on his body since he was a child. When he was thirteen, one slightly raised mole that became irritated when he played sports had been shaved. About three years later, another dermatologist saw this mole and, given its dark color, uneven border, and large size, recommended a biopsy to be sure it wasn't cancerous. When Jonas went back for the results, the chief resident sat him down for some bad news. He said that the mole showed a worrisome number of abnormal-looking cells and was cancerous. To make sure all the abnormal cells were removed, he needed to have a fairly extensive operation. This would involve removing some muscle around the buttocks.

Jonas was stunned. He was sixteen years old and had cancer! But he also had the presence of mind (future doctor in the making) to make absolutely sure the diagnosis was correct. So he asked whether there was any possibility that the suspicious-looking cells had been caused by the shaving done years before. The chief suspected Jonas was in denial and, somewhat nervous as all people are when delivering bad news, he flipped through the chart while expressing his certainty that the diagnosis was correct. The shaving, he told Jonas, had been done on the left side and the excision from the right. But no, Jonas said, they had in fact been from the same place.

The resident then saw that one notation had incorrectly stated where the mole was. The pathologist had found irregular cells on the sample surface and believed these to be the product of a natural process and therefore of medical concern. With the knowledge that the area had been shaved, the pathologist now reexamined the slide, took another sample from a deeper portion of the tissue, and concluded without any doubt that the sample was in fact normal. The proper diagnosis could only be made once they knew what tissue they were looking at.

The truth is that, in medicine, rights and lefts are everybody's nightmare. It's so easy to flip an X-ray and get mixed up, despite it being labeled. Before operating, surgeons, orthopedists, and others who may work on one side of the body will make signs that read left, right, or both. They will physically draw an X in magic marker on the place they plan to operate on, then check the consent form. And it better match up. If there's a discrepancy, it stops right there. All notes relevant to the operation—the booking (the operating room reservation), the doctor's note, the consent form (signed twice), the patient's approval, and nurse interviews (times three)—must all be the same.

In planning for a surgical case, I was taught always to write a doctor's note like the following: "I will do a right cataract because the patient cannot see in his right eye." I write this when I am sitting alone in my office, with no distractions, and concentrate on the words, etching them in my memory. The terms used in my field, OD and OS (that's *oculus dexter*, Latin for right eye, and *oculus sinister*, left eye) are easy to mix up. When the patient gets to the hospital, he will be asked, "What are you here for?" Thus the patient needs to articulate what needs to be done, which creates another opportunity to double-check that there aren't any mistakes.

In some hospitals, if the left and right don't match up, or if there's any question about it, the case is cancelled. I once oversaw a resident preparing for surgery. The nurse asked him specifically: "Which eye will you be operating on?" He didn't know. I asked him the same question. He was confused. I cancelled the case. When things were muddled like this, the doctor was not thinking clearly enough. This was elective surgery, not an emergency. Canceling the case was in part a lesson for the resident—such details are not to be taken lightly. With a senior physician, it's harder to cancel a case.

SWITCHED RESULTS: A CAUTIONARY TALE

A girl in my daughter's elementary school class, Sarah, complained of abdominal pain, and was thought to have appendicitis. Her parents took her to a fine pediatric surgeon. During surgery, he realized that it was an ovarian tumor, not appendicitis. The diagnosis was far from clear and would require more information from the pathologist.

The parents then took the child to a physician loosely affiliated with a fine institution for an opinion on treatment. This doctor started speaking directly to the child, warning her that she was going to lose her hair and telling her about the Make-a-Wish Foundation. Telling her, in other words, that she may well die. And all this before the parents had even agreed to the treatment suggested by this doctor. They then went to the main institution, where they received a very different treatment recommendation.

At this point, the mother, a physician herself, approached me and said that she didn't know what to do or whom to believe. I said, "Let's sort this out." I arranged a meeting with the director of pediatric oncology at Columbia-Presbyterian and the chief pediatric surgeon. The doctors had already discussed the case among themselves and searched the medical literature before the first meeting. The parents, without the little girl this time, brought the pathology slides and report and the blood test results to the meeting. I was hopeful; the pediatric surgeon in the group had participated in large-scale, multi-center studies, called national protocols, on just this type of tumor.

The group decided that the best plan was to watch the child with ultrasounds and CT scans over increasing intervals of time. First every week, then every month, and so on. At the same time, they monitored her with regular blood tests for a specific cancer marker. After a nerve-wracking year of watching and worrying, it looked as if the condition had stabilized, and the family tentatively returned to normal life.

The parents decided to go away on a brief vacation, their first break in a very long time. But a day before their trip, they received an urgent phone call: The blood test was sky-high. It looked as if the disease had come back full force. The parents thought the cancer had recurred. Forget the idea of any holiday. They thought that their child would quite likely die.

Meanwhile, the pediatric oncologist at Columbia-Presbyterian was urging a more measured approach. Rather than haul the child into the operating room or come to any conclusions in haste, he suggested that the test be repeated. His reasoning was that the four previous tests had been normal; it was unlikely that her condition would change to that extent so abruptly. They redid the test, and the results were once again in the normal range. Clearly the problem was not the disease, but the suspiciously abnormal test.

As it happened, this test was done at a suburban medical laboratory, as opposed to the hospital lab. As the problem seemed stable, the parents had wanted to start making things easier on the child. Someone at the lab had switched the girl's blood sample with someone else's. It was a simple mistake; someone had labeled the sample incorrectly. The girl was given a full metastatic work-up which revealed no problems, but for one very long week her parents had thought that she might die. And a less levelheaded surgeon may have quickly opted for surgery, which would have put the child at unnecessary risk.

This case is a reminder that when test results seem out of line, the test should be redone. Make sure you have the same set of constraints. The abnormal specialized test was done in a different laboratory. Sometimes complicated tests must be repeated in the same way in the same laboratory. It's like weighing yourself on the same scale over a period of days. Only the stakes here were a bit higher.

The final blow for the parents was that the suburban lab kept billing them for the egregiously mishandled test. Rather than adjusting the account appropriately, the billing department ultimately tried to put them in collections for it!

MEDICAL SLEUTHING AT WORK

A neuro-ophthalmologist at another hospital, Dr. John Martin, referred a patient to me. He was treating Alan Smith, a CEO businessman in his early seventies, for the loss of function of one of the nerves to the muscle in his eye, which caused Mr. Smith to see double. After some tests were run, including two CT scans to make sure Smith didn't have a tumor in his head, I was called in to consult. Correcting double vision is part of my specialty.

I treated the double vision and helped the patient deal with the headaches and depression that had resulted from the vision problem. After a few months he was better, and most importantly to him, able to get back to work. He was improving consistently and was almost as good as new. We determined that the probable cause was an infarct—a loss of blood for a short period of time, often described as a ministroke—to a small blood vessel feeding the nerve to a specific muscle.

Then, abruptly, another eye muscle went out of whack. His eyes, which had been going up and down, were now turning in. If my initial diagnosis had been correct, he should not have had the second round of trouble. This meant that either (1) this was a new and separate problem; or (2) we needed to rethink the first diagnosis.

As the picture had now changed, I suggested to Martin that we consider the possibility of ocular myasthenia, in which nerve transmission in the eye has been impaired (a disorder falling within his department). To have the first eye muscle problem is not uncommon. But two suggested a different and more unstable situation. I urged Martin to perform the tests for ocular myasthenia. The first test was called a Tensilon test, in which an injection of Tensilon concentrates the existing neurotransmitter by preventing it from being metabolized (breaking down). This essentially jumpstarts the process and allows you to see what is and isn't working. The results were borderline. The second test, electromyography (EMG), uses a needle to stimulate, and then assess, the muscle function of the eye muscle. This also came out borderline. Based on the tests, you couldn't say there wasn't a problem, but you couldn't say there *was* one either. Martin said,

"Let's treat it." The treatment for myasthenia involved significant doses of steroids.

Something about the pattern of the test results in conjunction with his eye muscle problem bothered me. Just bothered me. Enough so that I called Myles Behrens, M.D., a neuro-ophthalmologist at Columbia-Presbyterian and went through the patient's history. "Something is wrong here," I said.

Behrens said, "Martin is a fine doctor. It sounds like everything is okay."

"Take a look at the patient, as a favor to me," I said. He did.

So Behrens saw Smith for what turned out to be a two-hour exam and came up with a different diagnosis: a malformation of the blood vessels behind the eye. During the exam, the puzzle pieces started to fit together differently. Behrens heard a whooshing sound, which suggested a bruit—a net of blood vessels, something like a spider web, behind the eye. He ordered a CT scan to look behind the eye at the blood vessels—the first CT had been of the back of the head to check for tumors. This newest CT scan didn't show changes consistent with the web (an A [arterio] V [venous] malfunction) but didn't rule it out either. Because of his judgment and instinct, Dr. Behrens and his partner, Jeffrey Odel, M.D., persevered in this direction, which turned out to be right. It was an unusual problem, actually a variation on an unusual problem, but there it was.

I thought from the test pattern that maybe something was going on that we weren't catching. Also, I knew that the recommended treatment, steroids, was far from benign. In some people, steroids cause mood disturbances and other problems. But with my limited vocabulary in this specific area, I couldn't go past my intuition. In Behrens' subspecialty, neuro-ophthalmology, he would have access to a more specialized set of terms and assumptions, which would more precisely fit the situation. Sometimes picking up that something isn't right is enough to shift the diagnostic inquiry to a more productive line. Even if you don't have the answer. What I did was say: "Something's wrong. Dr. Behrens, you look at it with your diagnostic lens."

Meanwhile, Smith's symptom picture was getting worse. He could no longer move his eyes from side to side. The muscles of the eye were engorged, which suggested possible thyroid disease. Behrens asked Michael Kazim, M.D., the thyroid specialist down the hall, who said, "This is consistent with thyroid disease, but given the patient's history and symptoms, for me it doesn't fit." So the diagnosis still tilted in favor of the vascular web explanation. The process is like trying on different masks. You try one and then the other, and see which fits best. Every time you introduce another piece of information, the entire picture shifts. If they truly suspected thyroid disease, that would have suggested a whole group of other tests. The tiniest variation in observation can prompt an entirely new line of inquiry.

The suggested treatment for a malformation of the blood vessels around the eye can be best described as a special angiogram in which dye is injected into the blood vessels in the area behind the eye. To close them off, the doctor uses tiny wires within the guiding catheters to cauterize the abnormal blood vessels forming the web from within the blood vessel. It's a bit like pruning a tree, where you trim the smallest leaf on the skinniest, uppermost branch while working inward from the base of the trunk. A procedure such as this would be done by an interventional radiologist, someone who has experience with this technique.

When the patient heard what was involved, he flipped out. "Do I do it?" he asked me. "I could have a stroke from the treatment." I knew that the specialist who would perform the procedure was superb. Dr. Behrens had worked with him before and had good results. This, combined with his academic training and other credentials, suggested that he was the one to do it. I told Smith I would do it if it were I.

I was on vacation the day of the treatment, so I sent a medical student to watch. I told her she wasn't likely to see anything like this again. I also told her to tell me what happened—I really wanted to know!

The radiologist used a dye to light up the web of blood vessels. He found a massive web that went from one eye to the other. This explained 100 percent of the problem: why Smith had double vision, why his eye muscles and nerves were compromised. It also meant that the problem was treatable. Within twenty-four hours of the surgery, the swelling around the front of the eye had gone away, as had the headaches. And within three months, the muscle abnormality had reversed.

If we had not gone the extra step and pursued another diagnosis, Smith would have been taking steroids, which wouldn't have worked and might have caused serious side effects. Would Martin have ultimately come to the same conclusion? Probably, because the patient would have been getting worse and the problem more pronounced. But Behrens was able to catch it at an earlier stage. Had we waited until the steroids proved ineffective, Smith could have lost vision in both eyes. But nothing bad happened.

All because that first diagnosis didn't feel right.

DOING YOUR PART

To help the doctor make a correct diagnosis, keep these tips in mind:

✓ Keep of a log of your discomforts: when you're getting the pain, how long it lasts, in what setting (before eating or after eating, at the beginning or end of the day). Note anything that makes it better or worse: standing up or lying down, taking an aspirin, etc.

✓ Do not treat yourself before you talk to somebody. Medications can blur the diagnosis. If a physician sees you after someone has given you narcotics for pain or antibiotics, he or she is not getting a complete exam and may be missing important points.

✓ Keep track of your tests and records.

✓ Describe all symptoms bothering you and strong instincts you have about your condition. Even if they seem trivial, they could be important clues.

✓ Don't try to "outsleuth" the doctor. If you're convinced you know what you have, you can impede the discussion.

CHAPTER FIVE

Treatment

TREATMENT IS THE REASON YOU GO to the doctor; when you're sick, you want to be fixed. However, you can't really separate "treatment" from "diagnosis." Rather, there is a fluidity between the two. Your doctor might think the diagnosis has been nailed down. Upon embarking on treatment, however, it may become clear that the diagnosis needs refining. In actual practice, you end up bouncing between the categories of diagnosis and treatment because the diagnosis tells you one thing and your response to treatment suggests something else. This does not mean anything has gone wrong. It is a necessary step in the process of getting the care you need.

TREATMENT CATEGORIES

Some diseases are structural or mechanical, and require a surgical solution: taking something out (such as a cancer); putting something in (like a heart valve or artificial hip); putting things back together (replacing a joint, mending broken bones with cement, filling in crevices).

Infections—bacterial, viral, or in-between—are treated with medications. These include antibiotics, viral medications, medications for in-between infections, and antifungals.

Chronic diseases are treated with long-term replacement medications. Examples are Lipitor and similar medications for high cholesterol, oral or injectable insulin for diabetes, beta blockers, and other medications for hypertension.

DETERMINING THE APPROPRIATE TREATMENT

Treatment can be extremely simple: You have a mild headache and you take an analgesic. It doesn't matter which variety or which brand. It works, and you're cured.

Slightly higher on the pyramid would be a straightforward diagnosis with a tried-and-true treatment. Tests reveal a urinary tract infection, which is then treated with a simple antibiotic, and you're all done. Treatment can also be extremely complex: a juggling act of symptoms, side effects, and known statistics about the disease. Treatments like chemotherapy or radiation, for example, have to be carefully calibrated and tailored to you.

Determining the treatment is a multistep process, with essential questions that need to be answered along the way.

WHAT DO YOU HAVE? CHECKING AND RECHECKING THE DIAGNOSIS

Treatment and diagnosis are always intertwined. There is no such thing as "treatment" in isolation; the treatment is always specific to the diagnosis.

Let's say that you have a bad cold, the kind that leaves you curled up in bed emptying box after box of tissues. If it's bacterial in origin, an antibiotic will clear it up. If it's viral in origin, an antibiotic won't do a thing. You have a cold either way. But the question that needs to be asked is what kind of cold is it? The difference between the two has no effect on what you're experiencing, but it determines what you do about it.

This is why the diagnosis has to be double- or even triple-checked; if it's one diagnosis you treat it one way; if it's another you treat it differently. Once you make a diagnosis, you determine the treatment. And upon starting the treatment, you won't necessarily know that you've gone the right route until the treatment does—or doesn't—yield results.

Of course a cold is a relatively simple problem. The more complicated and serious the medical problem, the more difficult it may be to tease out the cause. Let's say you have pneumonia. It is diagnosed as bacterial pneumonia, and the doctor prescribes an antibiotic. You get better, but still aren't 100 percent. It turns out that it was a different variety of pneumonia, one that responds to a particular antibiotic. You know that now from the treatment. The treatment wasn't an exact cure for the diagnosis. It didn't quite do the job. So the doctor needs to modify the diagnosis in order to find the most appropriate treatment.

Now let's take another leap up the complexity scale and revisit Mr. Smith with the vascular web behind his eyes. At the outset, there was one diagnosis to explain the double vision—an infarct, or ministroke. That made sense at the time. Then he went on to have another episode of eye trouble. But this time, because different sets of eye muscles were affected, the double vision was side by side (like two pictures next to each other) as opposed to up and down (one picture on top of the other). The first diagnosis, the infarct, did not explain why this second problem had cropped up. This left us with a choice. We could regard this as a completely separate matter or try to find some connection between the two problems. This meant going back and reevaluating the original premise. It wasn't that we erred with the first explanation; it's that something new came up that rendered that diagnosis inaccurate.

Embarking on treatment before a diagnosis has been established is not wise—although it does happen. A friend of mine in her midsixties was having trouble seeing. She was thought to have presumptive temporal arteritis, a circulatory disorder that can cause a loss of vision. Her doctor prescribed steroids. This is the appropriate treatment for that illness. However, it hadn't been established that she *had* presumptive temporal arteritis. She wasn't tested for it until after she had begun the steroid treatment. And herein lay the trouble: Steroids can mask the underlying problem. So when the biopsy came back negative, there was no way to know whether this was because she didn't have the illness, or the steroids covered it up.

Premature treatment also interferes with diagnosis in cases where a person is given a narcotic for pain before anyone knows what that pain means. As uncomfortable as pain may be, its location and intensity are necessary clues to determine what's wrong with you. Absolutely, pain should be treated. But not before you know the cause.

WHAT ARE YOU GOING TO DO ABOUT THE PROBLEM? A MATTER OF JUDGMENT

Sometimes the diagnosis points clearly and unequivocally to a given treatment. But like the diagnosis itself, it is just as often a question of judgment. Doctors make the best treatment decision they can, based on the facts at hand. Even when the diagnosis has been determined and confirmed, the treatment may be up for grabs. This can be quite nerve-wracking, particularly when the stakes are high.

Such was the case with Sarah, the nine-year-old girl with the ovarian cyst. The physicians at each hospital examined her and reevaluated the laboratory report and pathology slides. There was little disagreement among the physicians as to what variety of ovarian cancer she had. But the array of recommended treatments was quite bewildering. Here's a kind of box-score rundown of the treatments that the various doctors suggested:

Doctor #1 said: Chemotherapy.

Doctor #2A (an oncologist) said: Surgery (a laparotomy—an abdominal surgery used to assess the stage of abdominal cancers), then chemotherapy, then a follow-up laparotomy to see how the treatment worked.

Doctor #2B (the surgeon affiliated with the oncologist) said: Surgery (laparotomy). If there's no problem, then no chemotherapy would be necessary.

Doctors #3A (an oncologist) and #3B (the affiliated surgeon) said: No surgery and no chemotherapy, but follow the patient with observation, CT scans, and blood work.

In sum, the choices were: (1) chemotherapy; (2) chemotherapy plus two surgeries; (3) surgery but no chemotherapy; (4) neither chemotherapy nor surgery.

Doctors #2B and #3B, you may recall, had been involved in a treatment protocol for this exact type of tumor and therefore had access to new information specific to the disease. They had found that the small subcategory of tumors that the little girl's fit into did quite well without surgery or chemotherapy. *And* that if the disease worsened or recurred, this type of tumor did respond well to chemotherapy. The treatment the family chose was *not* to treat, but to monitor carefully. Aside from the one false alarm, thanks to a mislabeled tube at the laboratory, she has been fine. That said, several physicians criticized the decision to forgo chemotherapy treatment. This demonstrates how, with the most complete data and most thorough consultations with the most reputable physicians, there can still be respectful disagreement.

In this case, the treatment itself wasn't complex; what *was* complex was deciding which treatment to pursue. Overwhelming though it may seem, the decision as to treatment must be made. You try to make the best decision you can—knowing that a less-than-optimal decision can have dire consequences. This isn't easy for anybody. It certainly wasn't easy for Sarah's family. They carefully looked at the data and read a very narrow interpretation of them. Of the five doctors they consulted, the first (who had offered chemotherapy as the only option) was not of the same stature as groups two and three. This made it easier to ignore what that first doctor said. And while groups two and three were of a comparable caliber, Sarah's parents felt particularly encouraged by the third group, and ultimately chose to follow their advice.

Sometimes the diagnosis, and therefore the treatment recommendation, is altered when new information comes into the picture. With Mr. Smith, one new element—the bruit, or web of blood vessels behind the eye found on a physical exam—changed everything. The treatment plan changed from waiting and monitoring (with the initial diagnosis, the infarct), to steroids (with the new working hypothesis, ocular myasthenia), to detailed vascular surgery behind the eye (once the bruit had been identified).

New data, and a new perspective, also prompted a complete about-face with my father's prostate treatment. Here's the story: My father had gone to a urologist for an enlarged prostate. The doctor watched him as his Prostate-Specific Antigen (PSA) test numbers continued to rise. Ultimately, he took biopsies. Evaluations of prostate cancer rely on the Gleason score, a 1 to 10 rating of severity, with 10 being the most severe. Based on the combination of the Gleason score and the PSA, the urologist did a metastatic workup. The CT scan showed an abdominal mass, which the doctor concluded was metastatic disease. (Note that the urologist had found a *mass*, not a *tumor*.) My father was told that he had metastatic prostate cancer. I heard this, panicked, and urged my father to see Mitchell Benson, M.D., a urologist at Columbia-Presbyterian who specializes in prostate treatments.

I called Dr. Benson, who told me: "Your father doesn't have metastatic prostate cancer." That was certainly nice to hear. I wanted to believe him. But he hadn't seen the patient. I asked him: "How do you know?"

He told me that he had looked at the laboratory tests the urologist had done. "The Gleason score was too low, and PSA was too low," he said. "We just did a big study, and no one with this combination of scores had metastatic cancer." Well, this was quite different from the first doctor's pronouncement. To make a treatment decision, Benson needed to look at the original biopsy results and blood tests. He scheduled my father for a needle biopsy of the abdominal mass.

The first doctor, a general urologist, had watched my father's PSA results rise from low to medium to high and done nothing. Then seemingly out of nowhere he announced, "Oh, you have a problem." Upon finding a mass on the CT scan he said: "I'll treat him and see if the mass gets smaller." To that, I replied: "But you don't know what it is," and took my father to another specialist.

Dr. Benson and the team at Columbia reviewed the films. I spoke at length with Dr. Jeffrey Newhouse, the radiologist who had collaborated on the study with Benson. Based on their research and the previous test results, both he and Benson believed that my father didn't have metastatic disease. Because they thought so, they looked even harder to find something. The team did a needle biopsy, a procedure done under general anesthesia in which the physician, guided by a radiologist, sticks a fine, long needle through the abdominal wall and into the mass. The needle retrieves cells from the mass, which can then be examined under a microscope.

What they found was not cancer but an enlarged lymph node. This radically altered the category of disease. The change in diagnosis also altered the recommended treatment. Certainly with a younger man and possibly even with an older man, metastatic prostate cancer would be treated with an aggressive surgery and chemotherapy regimen. What my father had would be treated differently: with radiation to make sure no abnormal cells spread.

The point is that a new diagnosis means new treatment. However, people often get impatient while a consulting physician reviews and refines the diagnosis: "Why is this new doctor asking these questions and ordering these tests? My doctor told me what I have!" They want to get on with the treatment, which to them means that they're going to get better. However, it's never a question of a treatment being good in and of itself, but whether a given treatment is right in the context of what you have.

HOW IS THE TREATMENT DONE? TECHNIQUES AND TECHNOLOGY

Once my father's problem was determined, the treatment was clear: radiation. However, the type and application of radiation varies. This was the next decision we needed to make. Dr. Benson recommended cone radiation, in which radiation exposure is limited to a very narrow field. At the time, only two hospitals in the city did this particular type of radiation. Fortunately, Columbia-Presbyterian was one of the two. Because we were in a good place, we were well-situated to get the right treatment. Had we been at another hospital, either (1) we might not have known about cone radiation and simply taken what they had; or (2) we might have sought out a radiologist who did cone radiation and gone to another medical institution. This was a time of great stress for us; it was nice not to have to switch hospitals midstream.

There are always variations in treatment forms and techniques. Treatments may look similar to the consumer, but have quite different ramifications for your health. It's a lot like the way you might use ingredients in cooking. With butter, the variety or even the brand you use depends on the recipe. In a sauté, you might use lightly salted butter, but for baking, you may choose sweet butter. Similarly, the intensity of a spice's flavor and its effect on the dish may change if you put it in at the beginning of the recipe or at the end. To take a medical example, a common variety of amblyopia is decreased vision in one eye and normal vision in the other. The treatment strategy is to use glasses with a prescription in only one lens to improve the weaker eye. The treatment also often requires putting a patch on the one good eye. However, there are alternatives (think sweet or salted butter). Sometimes an eye patch is used. Or an *invisible* eye patch. Or a medication that blurs the vision in the seeing eye. Or we'll do a combination of these things. There are often several ways to get the same result. These are the kinds of distinctions your doctors are making for you. It takes a high level of expertise to distinguish between treatments and to apply them; you need your doctor to help determine the best for you. Such subtleties are far from trivial. We can show you how to make sense of them.

Depending on the circumstances, the "how" part of treatment may be the most complex. For example, Mr. Smith's problem with blood vessels in the eye required truly state-of-the-art, NASA-plus-Star-Wars–level science and technology. As I explained in the last chapter, in this particular surgery, an interventional radiologist threads little wires into the tiny webs of vessels and cauterizes them. The problematic vessels disappear. On all levels, from the know-how to the technique to the equipment and support, this was beyond complex. Only a very few radiology subspecialists can do this.

Because the treatment is so new, I asked Behrens whether he had sent other patients to this particular radiologist for this or similar treatment. "Yes," he said. "The procedures went very well." So now when the patient asks me, "What do you think?" I can say, "My personal answer to you is that this is very new stuff. I have not seen patients through the process, but Dr. Behrens has, and he would have articulated any concerns he might have." "Yes," I conceded, "there is the risk of stroke." But if he didn't do it, he might have gone blind—and his condition was getting worse. If it were a family member, I would have said to do it. Knowing that boosted my comfort with this recommendation.

Treatments are continually evolving. When we look back a couple of centuries, we are appalled at the state-of-the-art medical treatments of the time, of which leeches and bloodletting are only two of the most flagrant examples. (Actually, in the field of plastic surgery, leeches are making a comeback.) Probably 95 percent of any contemporary doctor's treatment repertoire would not have been dreamed of even one hundred years ago. The pace of medical advancement has only quickened as technology continually creates new possibilities. The development of plastics through the space program and industry in the 1970s led to great improvements in medical technology. Plastic is everywhere in medicine: intravenous (IV) tubing, IV bags, and syringes to name just a few of the most ubiquitous. IV bottles used to be made of glass; you dropped one and it broke. That's no longer a problem. And advances in anesthesia opened the way to more sophisticated surgical treatments, as surgeons are now able to sedate patients long enough to perform such complicated operations. Today, computers are changing how medicine is administered from a distance. We can email CT scans and reports and have a discussion with someone across the globe in a moment's time.

I've seen incredible changes in treatment over just a few years. When I was in medical school, a child diagnosed with leukemia would die. Now, the vast majority will survive. Similarly, in the beginning of the AIDS epidemic, HIV was considered a death sentence. Now there's effective treatment. I recently saw a fifteen-year-old girl who was born HIV-positive, and she's never shown signs of the disease. We've made vast strides in once-complicated procedures such as fixing holes in children's hearts. This used to be major, invasive surgery. Now techniques have moved forward to allow for indirect treatment where, via an angiogram, the surgeon stitches between the two pieces in order to join them. The results have been amazing.

All sorts of razzle-dazzle breakthroughs are happening right now. New drugs and treatments are approved every year. Some have been approved in Europe and are awaiting approval here. A doctor may say, "I don't do that treatment, but you can go to

THE DOCTOR'S NEW ASSISTANT

Leeches are making a comeback. In a modern-science-meets-medieval-medicine scenario, leeches are now being utilized after certain surgical procedures.

In many areas of plastic surgery, especially when hands, fingers, or skin grafts are involved, the suturing must be very fine. There is always postoperative swelling—but no way to drain the extra pooling of blood and fluid.

This is where the leeches come in. A leech will drain the extra fluid or blood gently and delicately—without disrupting the surgical site. When a leech is "full," it is removed from the site and the next one is put in place.

And the best part? They don't hurt!

London for it." No matter how large the world may look to you, the patient, the world is a small place to today's physicians.

WHO DOES THE TREATMENT?
SPECIALISTS AND STRATEGIES

Often the doctor who makes the diagnosis will treat you. This could be a generalist, such as your internist. In other instances, you may be referred to another physician for treatment. Again, your diagnosis determines what subcategory of doctor will treat you. If you need highly specialized treatment for, say, your eyes, your diagnosis would point you in the precise direction. There are specialists who work on the cornea, others that treat the middle of the eye, and still others who deal with the back of the eye. As for the retina, two or three subgroups can handle that. If you have one disease you would see one person; if you have another one, you'd see a different person. A consumer may find it difficult to distinguish between these specialists. But each treats different diseases and specializes in a different type of treatment.

In many cases, "Who does the treatment?" is the pivotal question.

Last fall, Julia, a child in my son's class, missed a full week of school. I knew Julia's mother, a college placement advisor, and asked her what was going on. She told me that Julia had asthma and had a cold on top of it. She was having trouble breathing. She had seen the pediatrician several times, and the usual asthma medicine did nothing. On Friday, the wheezing was so bad that Julia's mother took her to the emergency room, where the ER doctor was only able to break the attack after three rounds of treatment. What really alarmed her mother was the look of fear in the ER doctor's face. Something was clearly wrong. Ten days after the problem started, Julia was better, but still not well. Her mother didn't know what to do.

As I heard this story, several red flags went up for me. Many of my patients take asthma medication, and I knew how serious a condition it can be. It can change quickly, like flash fire. I responded to the mother's being spooked by the ER doctor's reaction; she said the doctor's face virtually turned gray. And to her frustration, her trusted pediatrician wasn't showing her a way out of the crisis. It seemed to me that the child was sicker than the mother had been made aware. I said, "I'm at Babies' Hospital. Is there anything I can do to help?" She said no.

I knew that, on an elemental level, she knew her child needed help. She had been staying home with her, despite this being peak time for college applicants. But she didn't know what her alternatives were. And she was reluctant to challenge her doctor.

Stop right there: When that little voice starts saying, "There's a problem!" listen to it. You're not wrong. There's nothing like doubting a trusted doctor to raise your own insecurities, but you've got to follow up on your doubts. If a treatment isn't working, then you need either (1) a different treatment approach, or (2) a reevaluated diagnosis. And when you're dealing with a problem like asthma, you need to shift gears fast.

I called Dr. Lynn Quitell, a pediatric pulmonologist at Columbia-Presbyterian, described the situation, and asked her whether she was available to see Julia in short order. She said she could see her the following day at 9:00 A.M. Then I called the mother back and told her that a pediatric pulmonologist would be able to see Julia the next morning. Would she accept the appointment? Ultimately, she decided to trust me and took Julia to see the specialist. (This was much the same way that I had trusted her with my daughters' college decisions.) And she was scared. The next morning, Dr. Quitell gave Julia steroids and modified her asthma medicine. Within three hours, Julia's condition greatly improved. Within twenty-four hours, she was completely better.

In this case, the crucial step was getting Julia to the specialist. The girl was in trouble, the mother was nervous, and the pediatrician was sitting on his hands. The bell went off—the ER doctor broke the attack only with great difficulty and betrayed a suppressed panic—sending the message: "Do something." Here, I intervened and helped route the mother to the appropriate specialist. However, there are several different options she could have used to reach a similar place on her own. These could work for you, too:

Call the referral line of a major medical center. The operators at the medical center there are trained to handle the request and will know to route you to the referral line even if you don't know the precise name of it. The doctor's referral network provides a standing resource. Once Julia's mother said, "I have a child with asthma," the person on the line would direct her either to a pediatric pulmonologist or a pediatric allergist. There is a large overlap between the two. I chose a pediatric pulmonologist because asthma was the sole problem. If, by chance, the mother called the wrong doctor, the secretary in that office could say, "Dr. X doesn't handle such cases, but you could try Dr. Y."

Call a children's hospital in her area. The operator at the children's hospital, which by definition only handles children, would plug her into the network, directing her to the pulmonary specialists on staff.

Zero in on the hospital she wanted to use. Then, she could have called the secretary of the chairman of pediatrics there to ask for help. The office would be very accommodating and get her where she needed to go.

Search by specialty. Julia's mother didn't know that "pediatric pulmonology" was the appropriate subspecialty. How could you determine what specialty you need? First, you know you're dealing with a child, so you know you need a pediatric specialist. You can call the American Board of Pediatrics and say that your child has asthma. The person there will make the jump to pulmonology or allergic medicine and give you a group of names in your area. This is a good place to start.

Note that in this case, some allergists are good at treating asthma. However, *all* pulmonologists are good at treating asthma. What you can do: When you call to make an appointment, question the secretary and ask if the physician deals with asthma predominantly or exclusively. When you have the choice, go with the person with the most experience in your particular problem.

Julia and her mother may not have found their way to Dr. Quitell specifically, but they would have found a competent, qualified physician with similar results.

You may need to change venues for treatment. In order to get optimal care, Julia had to leave her original doctor. Similarly, there are times when you might need to move to another hospital. As always, you want a reputable, board-certified physician to treat you, and you want the treatment done at a quality place where all physicians—the ones that treat you directly as well as those behind the scenes—are high caliber.

Individual doctors have their strengths. The flip side to that, unfortunately, is that most doctors have their weaknesses, too. When you're dealing on the level of highly specialized experts,

AROUND THE WORLD

Today, the question of who "treats" you needn't be limited by geography; doctors around the world can assist in a patient's care. Here are two examples of twenty-first-century telecommunications doctoring that I've participated in:

* A two-day-old newborn in Dubai, the child of U.S. diplomats, came down with meningitis. This is a serious disease with potentially dire consequences; in a baby so young, this was especially terrifying. The parents decided against airlifting the child out of Dubai. The baby's grandparents, understandably frantic, called their internist here in the States, and the internist called me. I gave him the names of two pediatric infectious disease specialists at Columbia-Presbyterian. Almost immediately, one of them spoke with the internist, expressing his willingness to speak with the doctor in Dubai. The doctor in New York shepherded the child's case, telling the doctor abroad which tests to take, what to look for, and how to treat the baby. The child pulled through, much to everyone's great relief and joy.

* The son of a diplomat stationed in Bosnia had an accident. A sharp stick had gone straight into his eye. His aunt in Connecticut calls her obstetrician/gynecologist at Columbia-Presbyterian, who calls a pediatrician friend, who calls me. I learn that the boy has been airlifted to Wiesbaden, to the excellent U.S. military hospital there. I am about to call my friend at Walter Reed, the top military hospital in Washington, when I learn that the people in Wiesbaden have sent him to an eye clinic nearby. I had heard about the superb local clinic, but didn't know individual doctors by name. A retina specialist down the hall from me had grown up in Germany and went to medical school there. He would know the people. My colleague called the aunt and was able to reassure her that the doctors treating her nephew were very good and were in fact the senior faculty. Had that not been the case, the family would have known which doctors to request.

Medicine is a small, interconnected world.

you may need to come up with a strategy that gives you the benefits of specialized treatments with the security of personal care.

Jenny, the sister of a close friend, has multiple myeloma, a blood cancer. This is a serious, difficult-to-treat illness. She picked a doctor in New York who was known for dealing with this condition, undeniably the expert in his field. As to his knowledge and competence in dealing with the most intricate manifestations of the disorder, no one had any question. On a more practical, logistical level, however, his solo practice was bursting at the seams; he had no partner and limited office support.

Jenny went to the hospital for a stem cell transplant. Stem cells are the undifferentiated cells that are precursors to all the various cell types in the body. They are the basis for all human cells. The treatment involves wiping out the patient's bone marrow and then inserting stem cells from a donor or the patient. The hope is that these will grow as normal cells. This is an exceedingly risky procedure; during vulnerable parts of the process, getting so much as a cold can be fatal. Right at the outset, there was an infection at the IV site. This could have been avoided. But once it happened, they had to cancel the procedure. Jenny couldn't get the stem cells at that time because her physician had tripped over the easy steps; she lost time in a situation where she had none to lose. She also got an infection—this in somebody already sick and possibly dying.

The family was in an uproar. They wanted Jenny to change doctors, but found themselves faced with a dilemma: This guy was the best in the field and, arguably, the only doctor around with knowledge and experience in Jenny's specific illness. After much discussion, they opted to go with a physician with less expertise. The second doctor, they reasoned, would at least be proficient at the basic procedures. No matter how brilliant the guru specialist may be, if he can't manage the easy, more straightforward aspects of treatment, then his care is truly dangerous.

Jenny, however, didn't want to switch doctors. She liked the guru specialist and felt, with his erudition and insight, that he was the person to help her. So this is the win-win compromise they made: they found an A-plus internist at the medical center where the guru specialist practices. This way they can interact with the internist, who will watch out for Jenny and track her treatment. They had at times had trouble getting through to the expert. Now the internist can act as an intermediary. If there's a problem, they can speak to the internist, who, as a colleague, the guru will listen to.

WEIGHING THE PROS AND CONS

Before giving your okay to a treatment plan, you need to consider any possible downsides. Find out any potential negative consequences there could be to (1) accepting treatment; and (2) not accepting treatment. This allows you to weigh your options in a more informed way.

For example, what happens if you have acute appendicitis, and you don't have your appendix removed? Answer: You could get peritonitis and maybe die. Well, that's a good reason to go with Treatment Plan A and have an appendectomy. Or say you're dealing with bacterial meningitis. Without treatment, you could suffer brain damage with altered mental function and maybe go deaf. Suddenly the antibiotic doesn't look so bad.

Treatment decisions are less clear-cut when the treatment itself is difficult. The best-known example is chemotherapy. But if a course of chemotherapy would help you beat the statistical risk of cancer or recurrence, you do it. It's a numbers game, and you play the numbers as best you can. This is why the more precise the diagnosis—the most exact subcategory of disease you can pin down—the better able you are to determine the treatment. You need to know that you're comparing apples and apples without an orange or two sneaking in.

Sarah's family, for example, decided not to actively treat her ovarian cyst. They knew that each of the treatments offered had downsides. Chemotherapy is arduous, uncomfortable, and carries many side effects. It may be particularly disruptive for a young child, who would have to be taken out of school and activities for treatments. Surgery always brings risk and discomfort, and would also upset the child's daily life. The downside to *not having* the treatment, however, would be minimal, with no discomfort. They believed from the research that if she were to have a recurrence, that particular type of tumor would respond to treatment. That is why the treatment they chose was watching the child while keeping the more aggressive treatment, chemotherapy and surgery, in reserve. Time would tell if they had made the correct decision.

The essential knowledge in this case was which subgroup of tumor she had. If you looked at the group as a whole, chemotherapy appeared to be the treatment of choice. But if you followed her specific type of tumor, a high percentage of the latest group of children seemed to do fine without it.

CHECKING UP ON TREATMENT

How do you know if the treatment is effective? With an acute infection, you will know immediately. The antibiotic generally kicks in on the second or third dose, so within twenty-four to thirty-six hours you will know that you're on the mend. It will take a longer time to feel fully better, but you've got a start. Still, you will have to take the medicine the complete seven- or ten-day course.

In the more complicated cases, as with cancer, you may not know for five years whether the treatment has done its job. Linda, who had the bilateral mastectomies, is still waiting to see if she is cured from her cancer. In a few years, it will become clear whether she needs to undergo chemotherapy or radiation treatment. And if she does require further treatment, her physician must still determine the interval of treatment and which drugs and doses to use. All of these decisions are exceedingly complex.

Some diseases have a more predictable pattern. A cataract is a good example. First, the lens in your eye starts to get cloudy. You have trouble seeing. You have surgery to remove the cataract and, voilà, you're all better. It's nearly always just that straight-forward. If you wait too long before treatment, however, your eyes can become inflamed and you might require a more complex procedure.

Certain chronic conditions ebb and flow; that's part of their disease pattern. As a result, illnesses like gallbladder disease, inflammatory bowel disease, and arthritis present differently at different times. One day you're very uncomfortable, and the next day you're better. A physician might offer different advice depending on the day because the condition appears so radically different. If it looks severe, the doctor might suggest aggressive treatment. If it's milder, the advice may be "wait and see." In such instances, you need to establish the range of the problem before you settle on a treatment plan. To do this, you may need to see your physician several times so that he or she can observe your symptoms over a period of time. A good specialist will know that a particular disease has this varying picture and take this into consideration.

It's a lot like trying to buy clothes when your weight fluctuates widely because of water retention. What size do you wear? Well, it depends. With a fluctuating illness, a lot depends on the doctor and the patient's level of tolerance. Some physicians are quick to treat, others more conservative. You need to find somebody in sync with you. Again, these are matters of judgment. If, say, to preserve your joints you need to be treated energetically, there's no question. Other times, however, the issue is balancing discomfort and side effects. A physician may be reluctant to put you on a higher dose of medication unless you're uncomfortable most of the time. You might have a bad day and get through it. But if every day is a bad day, you will need more treatment.

In order to treat you effectively, your doctor will need to know if this is the beginning of a new pattern or a mere blip on the screen. With such conditions it may be fruitful to keep a diary. A good doctor can help you do this.

When it comes to pain and discomfort, treatment patterns vary from doctor to doctor and patient to patient. And the standards evolve over time. A fine example of this is treating young babies for pain. For several decades it was thought that infants didn't feel pain the way older children did and that any benefit would be outweighed by the pain medication's side effects. Then research showed that when newborns had their skin pricked or were given painful treatment, their heart rate and blood pressure jumped. That was their response to pain. This confirmed what many people intuitively believed: Yes, babies feel pain. Now physicians are far more aggressive in treating pain in newborns.

It was the same with cancer patients. Physicians used to low-ball pain medication; they were reluctant to overmedicate and leave the patient drug-dependent or sedated. Again, that's changed. In part, this was because there are new medications, derivatives of the more severe drugs, that cause fewer problems. Also, physicians have learned how to fine-tune the treatments to avoid over-sedation or dependence. But another reason is philosophical. Physicians have come to believe that some levels of discomfort warrant high-level narcotics and that we shouldn't be afraid of easing the pain. Today there's an entire specialty for pain management within the larger field of anesthesiology. There are different tactics for lower back pain, whole body pain, bone pain, and so on.

With chronic disease, find out what simple things that you, as the patient, can do to make yourself better. These include lifestyle changes: quitting smoking; losing weight if you need to. Sometimes you can make lifestyle changes on your own. Sometimes you struggle with them, which can be infuriating. However, you can always ask your physician for additional help. That's part of treatment.

CHAPTER SIX

Second Opinions

M ANY PEOPLE HAVE THE WRONG IDEA about second opinions. There's a sense that it's a means of "checking up" on your doctor, and that if you really trusted your doctor you would simply do what he or she says. But this is not true. A second opinion simply means consulting another doctor for a diagnosis and/or treatment recommendation for the same problem. As we've discussed, many medical decisions come down to a matter of judgment, and doctors may legitimately arrive at different conclusions about the same case. Another doctor looking at a situation may bring a new perspective to it.

An elderly relative of mine went to her general surgeon complaining that her belly was oddly large. She was told that she had an unusually large hernia down the middle of her belly. A hernia means that the contents of some organ or area protrudes through an opening, allowing the contents to come through. You can think of it as a pillow that has a tear and the stuffing is coming out. Usually they are "femoral" (in the groin area, typically a man's scrotum), or "inguinal" (at the fold between the lower abdomen and the leg).

The surgeon informed her that this would require surgery to repair. As I've become something of the family clearinghouse for medical crises, she called me and told me about it. She was fully prepared to have surgery, but she wanted me to know. I said, "I don't know what you've got," and suggested that she get a second opinion before choosing to have surgery. Her situation seemed odd; she looked seven months pregnant, and it seemed peculiar to have a hernia in that area. I am not a general surgeon, but I did know of someone who could give her some answers.

I gave her the names of two general surgeons, one at St. Lukes-Roosevelt, a Columbia affiliate, and the other at Columbia-Presbyterian. Second-Opinion Doctor #1, Dr. George Todd (who had been at Columbia-Presbyterian and was now chief of surgery at St. Lukes Roosevelt), disagreed with her original doctor, saying that an operation to treat it would be unnecessary surgery. Furthermore, he disagreed with the diagnosis. In this case, her abdominal muscles were lax and her belly bulged out. But there was not a tear in the sac or muscles, as there would be in a hernia. In Dr. Todd's opinion, there wasn't anything to fix.

She had trouble believing this, so I told her to go to Second-Opinion Doctor #2, Dr. John Chabot. Dr. Chabot agreed completely with Dr. Todd. There was no hernia, and no reason to do surgery. Now, instead of one doctor telling her to have the operation, she had two out of three telling her not to. The problem, it seemed, was merely cosmetic. And at her age—she was in her late seventies—surgery would have put her at risk for other problems.

THE IMPORTANCE OF SECOND OPINIONS

We've seen the impact of second opinions in several instances from the last two chapters: Alan Smith, the man with the web of blood vessels behind his eye; and Sarah, the young girl with the ovarian cyst, to name just two. If they had not sought out additional viewpoints, they would not have enjoyed the same fortunate outcomes.

Alan Smith would have been on steroids, and the treatment that saved his sight would have been delayed—perhaps at the cost of irreparable damage. Sarah would have been on a harsh chemotherapy regimen—perhaps unnecessarily. As a patient, it is in your interest to gather opinions from different physicians. In determining the most appropriate diagnosis and the most effective treatment, you—and any doctor treating you—need a broad base of information to draw from.

CONFIRMATION OR DIFFERING OPINION

If, as often happens, the second physician ends up confirming what the first doctor says, this is far from a waste of time. Getting verification for one doctor's opinion is important. When you accept a doctor's assessment and recommendations, you are betting the farm that his or her pronouncement on your case is correct. This assessment affects all subsequent treatment. So if having two different opinions is helpful, in that it gives you a choice or suggests where you might need more information, having two *agreeing* opinions is superb; you can now proceed to treatment with greater confidence.

Another common myth about second opinions is that, in seeking one, you will somehow offend your doctor. You can safely drop that idea. If your doctor takes umbrage at your seeking a second opinion, I would question that doctor's judgment. No doctor should be more invested in being right than in the patient's welfare. Good doctors know their limitations. Responsible doctors appreciate the wisdom of medical collaboration. Far from being insulted, a fine doctor will welcome another voice, for in medicine two heads are often better than one. This is particularly true when the conclusion isn't clear-cut and the doctor has already been weighing different possibilities.

A second opinion is not questioning the honor and dignity of your well-intentioned M.D. Its purpose is to reevaluate the puzzle pieces and make sure they are assembled in the correct way so as to reach the same diagnosis or a different one. If it is indeed a different one, you must figure out why. Everything follows the diagnosis. You can have the greatest, most advanced treatment in the world, and it won't work if you're depending on the wrong diagnosis.

Don't let a feeling of loyalty to your doctor deter you from pursuing a second opinion. Remember: Your health is at stake. You are the consumer. Sy Syms, a legendary clothes salesman in the New York area, uses this mantra: "An educated consumer is my best customer." Ditto for medical care. Getting a second opinion enhances your knowledge about your condition, which makes you be a better consumer. This is to everybody's benefit.

In this day and age, second opinions often serve as a check against unnecessary surgery. There's a cultural stereotype of the scalpel-happy surgeon who wants to build an addition or buy a yacht on the bounty from his operations. But this is not so. In deciding upon a treatment, the decision *not to* operate is more difficult to make than the decision *to* operate. This is not a matter of drumming up more business. Rather, it reflects a very real desire to help people. A high-level, ethical surgeon prizes his judgment, honor, and professionalism above all else, but it's always easier to tell someone, "I'll fix you." It's harder to say no.

Physicians can respectfully disagree about the need for surgery. As we've seen, someone else might look at the very same puzzle pieces and say, "No, I don't think surgery is necessary." I recently conducted a second opinion for a child whose doctor recommended surgery. My exam yielded numbers that did not point to surgery. The first doctor's did. That did not mean that he is a lesser doctor or even that he was wrong. The child's parents asked me, "What is the downside of not doing the surgery?" Nothing, I told them. We can hold off on surgery, and if the situation gets worse, they still have that option. Surgery may in fact be needed, but I didn't see that at the time.

Similarly, the general surgeon who suggested that my relative have abdominal surgery wasn't an incompetent doctor. He had a dissenting view about a troublesome, not very clear, symptom picture. He was trying to help her. In many situations in medicine there is no "right" answer, but you still have to make a judgment. It's not black and white, but shades of gray. Physicians may see the patterns differently and thus come to different conclusions. Why did the Constitution institute a bench of nine judges on the Supreme Court? It's the same thing.

A COMPLETE REEVALUATION

Frequently, the second-opinion doctor will confirm the original doctor's diagnosis or treatment plan. But in order to concur with a diagnosis, all the factors need to be checked over again. This isn't a simple grant of approval, as in, "Does the next guy like my dress?" This is a matter of ensuring the right course of treatment. To arrive at a conclusion, one needs a lot of puzzle pieces. You have to have those pieces and they must fit together.

Medical consumers need to understand that this is part of the process. The original conclusion is an *assumption* on the part of the first doctor. It is not a given, it is not written in stone. It is a working hypothesis, no more. You go to someone else to verify that same conclusion. It is not an extra thing.

The initial doctor may say, "This is what you have," and send you to the person who treats that problem. But you need to know if indeed you *have* what the first doctor says you have. Verification is part of the medical care package.

The bottom line is this: Once you make a diagnosis, you commit yourself to a course of treatment. Once you start treatment, you don't always know if you're heading down the right road. If a treatment doesn't work well, is it because the antibiotic isn't effective or the wrong antibiotic was chosen? That's why second opinions are so important.

YOUR SECOND OPINION APPOINTMENT

✓ Request that the doctor send a report to you *and* your primary care physician. Find out what other information would help the consulting doctor. The more relevant information you come in with, the better.

✓ Bring somebody with you. You want to get as much of what the expert says as possible. You need another person to hear what the physician says because you're each likely to hear different things.

✓ Do your best to make sure that you understand what the expert says. Ask the doctor for as detailed an explanation as you need. Sometimes there's a nurse or assistant who can devote more time to this. In cases where the diagnosis is difficult to explain—which is often—it can be helpful for the doctor to draw the condition for you.

✓ If what the consultant says differs from what you have heard before, ask how he or she came to this conclusion. Knowing the doctor's train of thought may help you understand his or her perspective, and also help you explain it to your primary care doctor should you discuss it.

Sometimes the second-opinion process involves another physician taking a fresh look at the data that are already there. The doctor offering a second opinion may not have to reinvent the wheel. However, he or she may need to refine and add specifics.

You may ask the second physician, for example, to reevaluate your tests. Before the appointment, you can make photocopies of your X-rays, test reports, and so on. Many people are intimidated by these tests; there's a mystique about them, as if they were some kind of mystic oracle. But they belong to you, and you should get the full benefit of them. The second-opinion doctor may look at an X-ray and say, "I don't see that in this picture," or, "I see something else in the X-ray." They may suggest that you redo a test. Or maybe the test is meaningful in a different way now because you are at this point considering a diagnosis that would take those specific tests into account.

Often, if you back up the decision tree, the conclusion isn't as finely tuned as it should be. Or, there may have been a reinterpretation of a test made down the line, perhaps in the pathologist's reading of a surgical biopsy or an interpretation of an X-ray. Or sometimes a consulting physician is simply better than the primary doctor at explaining certain aspects of a medical condition or treatment to a patient.

WHEN TO GET A SECOND OPINION

You need to get a second opinion when:

The diagnosis is unclear. As we've seen, tests can be inconclusive. You would do well to see a physician with another frame of reference to help you get a handle on exactly what the problem is.

The diagnosis is serious. When you have a serious diagnosis, it can be difficult to grasp its magnitude. You will want another physician to confirm the diagnosis and to recommend treatment. A consulting physician may also have had similar cases from which to draw further insight.

Your doctor suggests surgery. When one doctor regards surgery as the best or only answer, another doctor may see other treatment possibilities. You want to be sure that surgery is the best approach before you consent to it. Many insurance companies will require a second opinion before surgery.

The course of treatment is unclear. Even when the diagnosis is clear, the treatment may not be so straightforward. Before you jump into an arduous or debatable course of treatment, you'll want to hear out other experts and learn about other options.

Your current treatment is not yielding results. Like anyone else, physicians can get in an intellectual rut and fail to see other possibilities. Or, he or she might be tied to a particular approach (as in, "let's see what happens"). If it seems as if your condition hasn't improved in a long time, let your doctor know that you are not satisfied with how things are progressing and suggest that another more specialized physician might offer a fresh perspective or second opinion. Your doctor should be able to suggest a specialist to consult. If not, you might want to seek one out on your own.

You want to evaluate how your treatment is working. After a period of time, you may want a reality check on how your treatment is progressing. For example, you may be wondering if a more (or less) aggressive approach would be more productive for you right now. A second opinion could (1) affirm the current strategy's effectiveness; or (2) offer suggestions to enhance your treatment.

Something has happened to jar your confidence in your physician. If you're not comfortable with your doctor's care or have reason to question his diagnostic or treatment decisions, don't let your doubts fester. A second opinion may reassure you about your doctor. Or it may confirm your misgivings and give you ideas of how to change direction. In either case, seeing another doctor can give you the vocabulary with which you can express your concerns directly to your doctor.

WHEN TWO ARE NOT ENOUGH

Sometimes two opinions are not enough. If you have consulted two physicians and their conclusions are miles apart, you should look into a third opinion. If their conclusions are inches apart and the difference will help determine your next step, consider a third opinion. If you want a tie-breaker and your problem isn't urgent, you can spread them out over time. This way you're not seeing three doctors in the same week.

Choose your consultants to cover as much ground as possible. For instance, find doctors from different practices, as doctors within a group practice often have a similar approach. Also, consider talking to doctors of different ages. A young doctor might be up on the latest treatments. However, an older doctor is likely to have more experience.

DON'T RUSH INTO ANYTHING: MAKE TIME FOR A SECOND OPINION

One day I called my Uncle Herbie to say hello and my aunt informed me that he was scheduled for a tonsillectomy at a local hospital in two days. Aunt Lucille said they hadn't wanted to bother me, but she was actually quite anxious about it. On top of everything else, I wasn't enamored of that particular hospital and was not thrilled by the prospect of him having surgery there.

PAYMENT

Check with your insurance company in advance to see how you should handle second opinions. Most insurance companies will pay for a second opinion. Some require it, and, in certain cases, won't reimburse you for surgery if you *don't* have it. (In the last several years, this has been the case for hysterectomies.) However, many will not pay for repeat tests. Make sure that any tests are forwarded to the appropriate consultant so that you won't be charged for duplicate tests. Also, while an insurance firm may reimburse for a third opinion, some will only do so if the two previous opinions have conflicted. Rules keep changing from year to year, even within the same insurance network. But as I've said before, don't let this stop you from pursuing the treatment you need. It is a vital investment in your health and well-being.

Apparently, they had gone to see their internist because my uncle's voice was hoarse. They were planning a trip to the Far East and wanted to make sure he was okay. The internist sent them to an ear, nose, and throat specialist who poked around in his throat and found what he described as some kind of mass on one side. The doctor said that he didn't know what the problem was, but thought the tonsil on that side should come out.

My aunt was terrified that Herbie had cancer and was going to die, scared enough that neither of them second-guessed the doctor's suggestion. But it didn't sound right to me. First of all, there had been no CT scan of the area, no MRI, no needle biopsy—any of which could have provided important information if a tumor was suspected. Even if there was a growth, it was very odd to remove the tonsil in an eighty-one-year-old. And in any event, simply removing the tonsil without a diagnosis would not have been the right answer. This is true for anyone, but for someone his age in particular any surgery needs to be considered carefully.

There are ENT doctors who are head and neck cancer specialists; I knew that their approach to his situation might have been different, no doubt more precise. I told Uncle Herbie that he had to go see another ENT. He agreed, so long as he could get an appointment within the next few days. Otherwise, he was going to have the surgery to get it over with before the trip. There was no way to reason with him about this; the trip was non-negotiable. I contacted the department of laryngology at Columbia-Presbyterian, and the first appointment I could get was with the head of the department, Lanny Garth Close, M.D. Anyone in the department would have been fine, but it's always nice to have the top dog.

Dr. Close agreed that the first doctor's verdict was strange, as eighty-one-year-old men tend not to have problems with their tonsils. He ordered a CT scan to make certain that the area was okay and that there weren't any other masses that he could neither feel nor see. He said he wasn't certain what Uncle Herbie had, and that he wouldn't operate except as a last resort. Basically, the first doctor said: (1) The diagnosis is unknown; (2) I haven't done an evaluation; and (3) let's cut it out. Dr. Close said: (1) I don't know what you have; (2) let's evaluate it; and (3) let's watch it. That made better sense to me. Uncle Herbie was happy; he liked the doctor because he was Texan and, like him, wore cowboy boots (the fact that I respected him and that he chaired a renowned medical department aside). He put my uncle on antibiotics and told him to come back after the trip.

Which they did. The trip was wonderful and they were glad that they didn't have to cancel it or be inconvenienced. The swelling didn't change, but it ceased to be a problem. The other fellow had been in a rush to operate—and would have, had I not insisted on a second opinion.

The moral of this story: SECOND OPINIONS ARE CRUCIAL. The moral within the moral is don't allow yourself to be hustled into surgery *without* a second opinion. Incomplete information can lead to a hasty response. Here, the first doctor seemed to want to do surgery to make up for the lack of a diagnosis. But that would have meant unnecessary surgery in a patient in his eighties. Also, the invisible doctors, the anesthesiologists and pathologists, were marginal at the hospital in question. With such a procedure, these are as important, if not more important, than the ENT. And beyond that, *had* it been a malignant tumor, it would have been wrong to take it out that way because sometimes cutting out a tumor spreads cancer cells. So this doctor's attitude was dangerous in several ways.

Oh, and one other lesson from the story: Your body takes priority over any trip—Uncle Herbie notwithstanding.

WHOM TO CONSULT: SPECIALISTS AND GENERALISTS

You need somebody who has the vocabulary of the disease in question. The higher you go up the specialist ladder, the more precise the language becomes. Most diseases are common; any competent doctor will be able to discuss these problems with some fluency. But not everyone can make the fine distinctions among variations of less common problems—distinctions that may determine the direction of your treatment. Since you don't want such distinctions blurred, you need someone who can speak to these finer points.

Before you make it to the specialist, the diagnosis might stay in that blurry zone for a long time. As a result, the problem doesn't get better. A good internist would catch this and suggest that you see someone with special expertise to examine you from a different perspective.

One condition that can catch physicians off-guard is arthritis in children. It's often not until the child goes to a pediatric rheumatologist, a physician specializing in muscular and joint problems among children, that the diagnosis gets nailed down. All of a sudden, it becomes clear that the problem isn't simply a bum knee. But before this happens, it may have been treated incorrectly for years.

When my daughter had knee pain that didn't abate, I knew enough to take her to a pediatric rheumatologist. Even though I see children with arthritis every day in my practice (as the disease can affect the eye), I didn't see the signs in my daughter. Of course, that's because she is my daughter and I was too close to the situation. In the exam, the pediatric rheumatologist said, "I see three other inflamed joints," noting the knee and both wrists. I had known she had a problem, but didn't know the degree of it. That is why I sought out a more specialized opinion: I knew the situation with my daughter's knee wasn't normal, and I wanted that to be explained to me.

We needed to go to the right person in order to identify the problem. A general orthopedist, who's not familiar with kids, might or might not have detected arthritis. It's less common in their practice, merely a small part of what they do, so they wouldn't always have the experience. There's overlap, but mainly their job is to know the bones. We needed the pediatric rheumatologist. A blood test, which finds markers for arthritis and autoimmune disorders in the blood, confirmed the diagnosis.

Now that we knew what she had, we needed a course of treatment. The specialist we saw suggested one approach, which involved using fairly aggressive drugs at the outset. We went to a second pediatric rheumatologist, who suggested starting with less aggressive drugs and then shifting to more aggressive drugs if needed. This wasn't a case of one doctor being right and the other wrong. They were both right. Rather, it was a question of style. We made the decision as parents, and chose the second specialist. This wasn't a clear or easy choice. Had I not had some understanding of the disease, we would have gone to a third person or, perhaps, checked back with our pediatrician for another viewpoint. As it happened, the less aggressive treatment worked for a long time, and when it ceased working, we stepped up the pace.

It's important to solicit second opinions from physicians at the same specialty stature. Once we had the diagnosis and wanted another perspective, we needed a physician with the same level of training and expertise in children's muscles and joints: hence a second pediatric rheumatologist.

One way to think about medical specialization is to compare it to something we've all had to deal with—auto repair. A generalist is the equivalent of a mechanic who handles all kinds of cars. A specialist would be someone who handles only Porsches. Say you go to your local mom-and-pop repair shop, and the mechanic says you need $1,000 worth of repairs. Unless you're a mechanic yourself, you don't know if this is reasonable and necessary. If you bring it to the dealership (the specialist), the people there will be more familiar with your car. They do maintenance and repairs only on the ten models their company puts out. Before you fix your car, you want to know exactly what's wrong. You don't want to fix five different parts if you don't need to. The person to ask is the one who knows your car the best.

In getting a medical diagnosis, the higher you go up the specialty ladder, the more familiar the doctor will be with exactly what you have. That's why going to a pediatric rheumatologist assured me a certain level of treatment. This is someone who does nothing but look at kids' joints all day, and will know all the various permutations of arthritis and other related diseases in children.

However, specialists have their disadvantages. They may tend to focus on the details that concern their area of expertise to the exclusion of more general problems—the proverbial missing the forest for the trees. As they are trained to look for the more unusual problem, they may be more prone to *see* the more unusual problem. In reality, the better the specialist, the more general knowledge they're likely to have. Correspondingly, the better the generalist, the more detailed their knowledge of specific problems. If you're lucky, you'll be able to pair them up: the specialist who sees the big picture with the generalist who knows a lot about many disease areas. Typically, you would work your way up the specialty ladder, not down. However, you can always check in with your primary care doctor. This is the person who knows you.

CRITERIA FOR CHOOSING A SPECIALIST

The criteria you use to choose a specialist for a second opinion are different from those for choosing a primary care physician. Personality issues are less of a factor. You're consulting this person specifically for his or her detailed expertise. A personable, understanding specialist is a fine thing to have, but you are not going to be developing the same kind of pivotal relationship that you have with your internist. Again, it would be nice if the specialist could explain things to you in a way you can understand. But in the absence of communication skills, your primary care doctor can be your go-between. With a specialized consultant, convenience is way down at the bottom of the list; you may in fact need to travel to a tertiary medical center for your second (or third) opinion.

Ideally, your primary care doctor makes the referral. When you self-refer, you need to do your homework. As with any doctor you choose, however, you will want to check the credentials and make sure he or she has received the appropriate certification.

The best way to select a specialist is to ask another physician, such as your internist, for two or three names. If you don't have a physician to ask, you can ask friends or start with a good medical center as a source of referrals. It's helpful to know a little bit about the consultant, including his or her medical orientation. Certain doctors are more aggressive than others in recommending surgery, for example. You can ask how your contact knows the physician in question. If you hear that your doctor sent thirty people to this specialist and everyone was happy, this is useful to know. You want someone to tell you that the person you are going to is honorable and that you can trust his or her judgment.

It's best to work through your primary care doctor—even if you make the actual choice of specialist on your own—for several reasons: (1) you will maintain your working partnership; (2) your internist can make the initial contact with the specialist for you, which may help you get seen sooner; (3) your internist can forward your records and may write a referral letter describing your problem; (4) your doctor can help prepare you for your appointment and suggest reading to acquaint you with the terminology the specialist may use; and (5) after the appointment, you can then "debrief" your internist, and he or she can help you determine your next step.

WHEN OPINIONS DIFFER

Sometimes when there seems to be a disagreement in a diagnosis or treatment recommendation, it's actually a difference in style. When you don't know the lingo, small discrepancies can look like huge differences. You need to have the second doctor explain exactly where they disagree. The doctor may be able to tell you,

"We agree about what you have, but disagree about what to do with it." Or, "We agree about what you have and what treatment you need, but prefer different variations of that treatment." The key points are: (1) the diagnosis; (2) the treatment; and (3) the style. In my field, I may prefer patching an eye for five weeks, while another pediatric ophthalmologist suggests only four weeks. On this level, it's a bit like cooking. Maybe one person uses rosemary and the other tends to use thyme. However, patients may think we're talking about completely different treatments.

As you compare opinions, you need to determine what the seeming differences actually mean. In many cases, the procedural differences—the nuances of care—matter far less than the doctor's competence. With cataract surgery, there's a new no-stitch technique, which is an advance from the one-stitch technique, which was itself an improvement over the several-stitch technique. So the surgeon who offers the no-stitch technique would seem to be the better choice. But I'd take the surgeon who is tops at the three-stitch version over the person who's learned the latest technique. We surgeons are effective salespeople; our conviction that we use the best techniques is part and parcel of our task. In general, the best surgeon does use the best, often more up-to-date techniques. But if an excellent surgeon gets fine results with a more traditional approach, then tried and true may be the best for you.

When the choice comes down to a matter of technique, you need to involve your primary care doctor in the decision. As the patient, you cannot judge nuances of technique and know what's most appropriate in your situation. What sounds good to the outsider may not reflect what's best. In many ways it's comparable to construction projects on your house: Sometimes you don't want the low bidder.

KNOW *ALL* OF YOUR OPTIONS

Often, an additional opinion gives you more choices. A few years ago, my husband consulted Paul McCormick, M.D., a fine neurosurgeon at Columbia-Presbyterian specializing in backs, about a long-standing lower back problem. Three years earlier, the same doctor had told Leonard that he wasn't ready for back surgery. By this time, the situation had deteriorated to the point that Dr. McCormick suggested an operation.

We decided that Len would go to two other doctors at two other hospitals, all three of whom specialized in backs. We went to the second person. He looked at the X-rays (we had made copies so they wouldn't need to be taken again). He offered the same diagnosis: spinal stenosis. This causes similar symptoms as a slipped disk, but in this case, rather than the disk, it's the bone that encloses the nerves of the spine and wreaks painful havoc. Basically, the nerve sits within a bony tree trunk. In this condition, the trunk is squashing the nerves. The bone around the nerve had to be opened to relieve this. Since the two doctors were in agreement, we did not consult the third.

So here we were: both doctors agreed on (1) what was wrong; and (2) what surgery was needed. Both were highly regarded practitioners working in top hospitals. But there were differences. First, Dr. McCormick personally saw his patients after the surgery; the other doctor would have his assistant see patients. Second, Dr. McCormick was a neurosurgeon, and the other was an orthopedist. From my perspective as a microsurgeon, I understood that to a neurosurgeon, the back is a large area. To an orthopedist, the bones of the back are small. Granted, that's my personal bias.

And finally, at Columbia-Presbyterian, anesthesia would be administered by a subspecialty anesthesiologist, a neuroanesthesiologist. This is someone who only does neurological cases, and therefore has more experience with this type of operation. It doesn't mean that the other is incompetent. But if you have the choice, and we did, your odds are better with the person who does this all the time.

We called our internist and asked what he thought we should do. He said, "My last several patients had excellent results with

Dr. McCormick." The orthopedist had good results too, he said, but Dr. McCormick follows his patients through the recovery. He verified my own leanings, but gave them a factual basis.

My husband, however, found this decision confusing. Both doctors were personable and had nice, helpful staffs. He could not distinguish between the two. I pointed out that with Dr. McCormick, the surgeon would follow him after the surgery. "But that's after the surgery," Len said. "It's the surgery itself I'm concerned about." No, I explained to him. That's *part of* the surgery. There were differences in the finer points of surgical technique. One surgeon would do a mini-incision and keep Len in the hospital for two or three days. The other would do a larger incision and Len would stay in the hospital for a week. These were not deal-breakers, but rather differences in technique between two very fine surgeons.

In cases where the decision isn't clear to you, your internist can help tip the balance—as he did for us. Len did have surgery with Dr. McCormick. Everything went smoothly, and any concerns he might have had afterward were taken care of. That was important to me, and I was glad that, between the two options, we had that choice.

PART THREE

THE INVISIBLE DOCTORS

FIVE WEEKS AFTER HE UNDERWENT quintuple bypass surgery, CBS *Late Show* host David Letterman, was back on the air. In characteristic fashion, his return monologue was interrupted by comedian Jerry Seinfeld, who walked onto the Ed Sullivan Theater stage and said, "What are you doing here? I thought you were dead."

To which Letterman replied: "I'm on CBS. I ain't dead. Why don't you go on home to your wife?"

It was exactly the way you expected Letterman to handle the situation: with a sharp retort, nothing sentimental or maudlin. But a few minutes later, the goofy comic visibly choked with emotion as, one by one, he brought on stage the personnel from New York-Presbyterian Hospital who performed the difficult operation and took care of him during recovery. This included the senior anesthesiologist, junior anesthesiologist, profusionist, OR nurses, Intensive Care Unit doctors, Cardiac Care Unit doctors, floor nurses, and home nurses, among others. The stage was positively overflowing. "It was five weeks ago today that the men and women right here saved my life," he said. The amazing thing is that this group went on to do a few more similar operations that very day. As they do day in and day out.

No one who was fortunate enough to see the show that February night in 2000 is likely to forget the poignant image of those fine doctors and nurses on stage, basking in Letterman's gratitude and the audience's applause. Nor are they likely to forget the touching picture of the hyper-ironic TV funnyman briefly fighting back tears as he sought to convey his very real and deep appreciation to them.

These images are worth remembering because Letterman grasped something that few people understand until they go through major surgery or face a serious illness: It takes a team of medical professionals to ferry you through your care. It's not just your doctor.

To the general public, these professionals stand in the shadow of the physician who tends to the patient. I call them the "invisible doctors."

And what you need to understand is that David Letterman didn't get great care because he was David Letterman. He got it because he went to a first-rate hospital—New York-Presbyterian—when his life was on the line.

You can, too. Once you know what to look for.

Much of medical care happens behind the scenes. When an internist sees patients in the office or a surgeon performs an operation, we know what's going on; this is visible to us. But what about that mammogram or X-ray that was taken? Who processes and evaluates it? Who determines your level of cancer risk when a biopsy has been taken? Who decides how long and how deeply you should be asleep during an outpatient surgical procedure?

Invisible doctors perform the essential, if unsung, tasks that accompany every aspect of medicine. The great paradox is that while the typical medical consumer knows little about their role, the invisible doctors are pivotal to the kind of care they receive. A further irony is that you can't pick them; they come with the package once you've chosen a hospital or physician. You pick your surgeon, and you get your anesthesiologist. And your pathologist, radiologist, and nursing staff. You can't say, "I'll take the anesthesiologist from here and the pathologist from there."

You may never even see these people. In fact, if you're lucky, you'll never even need them. But trust me on this: You want to know they are there if you do. In the course of your medical care, they will undoubtedly have an effect on your treatment. This is why it's so important to choose a good medical center. This is the only way to be sure that the invisible doctors who assist in your care are of high caliber.

This isn't only true of major surgery or tricky diagnoses. The big rule in medicine is that nothing is *ever* routine. Part of this is that nothing is routine if it involves you or someone you love; routine procedures are what they do on someone else. But this also acknowledges the need to be prepared for the unexpected. What at first seems "routine" can turn into something urgent or unusual quite quickly. That's why you want the best *at all* times.

TEAMWORK IS EVERYTHING

Many people say, "My doctor's great," and are reluctant to look further. Fine. Maybe your doctor is great. But have you thought about this: If you have to go to the hospital for bypass surgery or other major operations, who else will be working on you?

In the late 1990s, a group of Harvard Business School researchers conducted a fascinating study. A complicated new minimally invasive cardiac procedure was taught to eighteen surgeons and their teams. All came from highly regarded medical institutions. All received the same three-day training.

As the surgical teams began performing the new technique, the researchers followed their progress to study their learning curve. Everybody knew that there would be problems with the operations until they grew adept with the procedure. But it turned out that there was a huge gap in how well the various surgical teams did. Over the course of fifty cases, some teams were able to cut the time it took to perform the surgery in half. Others showed no improvement.

Atul Gawande, a surgical resident and staff writer for *The New Yorker,* cited this study in his excellent book *Complications.* He noted that one of the fastest-learning teams was led by a relatively inexperienced surgeon, while one of the slowest-learning teams was headed by one of the most senior and respected surgeons.

What was behind the less-experienced surgeon's success? Gawande recounts:

> "He made sure to pick team members with whom he had worked well before and to keep them together through the first fifteen cases before allowing any new members. He had the team go through a dry run before the first case, then deliberately scheduled six operations in the first week, so little would be forgotten in between. He convened the team before each case to discuss it in detail and afterward to debrief. He made sure results were tracked carefully."

In contrast, the more experienced and respected surgeon had different staff floating in and out each time. The surgeon himself was the only constant, while the people around him were substituted as if they were interchangeable parts.

And that's the point. These invisible doctors, as I call them, are *not* interchangeable parts. We, as surgeons, don't operate in a void. We need the nurses, pathologists, radiologists, anesthesiologists, and others. They make the surgeon look good. They make the surgeon *perform* well.

The Harvard Business School study wasn't about the surgeon. There's little question that while all the surgeons were superb, the senior, more respected doctor was a better, more technically proficient surgeon than the one who had been out of training a mere two years. In another context, the surgeon who has seen it all and done it all might have been the best for the job. But in this case—learning something new—the team counted as much as the surgeon. The surgeon was just one person. Granted, he was the leader, the general, the commander-in-chief. He performed the operation. He set the tone. But he needed good lieutenants, sergeants, corporals, and even privates.

Over the next few chapters, I'll be introducing you to some of the invisible doctors. But there are others: perfusionists (heart-lung bypass experts); ICU personnel; the engineers who maintain the complicated, life-saving machinery. These are your doctor's silent partners—silent from the patient's standpoint. They come and go, do their work with little if any patient interaction. The larger and more complicated your problem, the more you get into the invisible doctors' world. And you are entitled to know who is involved in your care.

CHAPTER SEVEN

The Anesthesiologist

YOU MIGHT THINK, "If I'm an otherwise healthy patient, why should I concern myself about the credentials of the person administering anesthesia?"

There's really only one reason: He or she can kill you.

I'm not being an alarmist here. It is a simple statement of fact that there's no way to know whether someone is going to have an unexpected—and potentially fatal—reaction to anesthesia.

It does happen. This is a rare occurrence in healthy patients. But if the right steps aren't taken immediately, significant airway difficulties can develop, which means the patient can't get air into his or her lungs.

This may be only one reason, but I think you'll agree that it's a pretty good one. But just as importantly, anesthesiologists can also save your life. They do it every day. The midair pirouettes they perform in the midst of complicated surgery allow great things to happen, things that were once unthinkable in the operating room.

The anesthesiologist's job is to maintain the patient's blood pressure and vital signs while keeping the person unconscious so that the surgeon can do what he or she needs to do. This has made new surgeries possible. This is every bit as important to the ultimate success of an operation as the surgeon's expertise. The skill involved in this balancing act of function and consciousness is simply astounding.

Anesthesiologists also play a key role in pain management. By using the right medications, they can keep patients sedated for a couple of days in the intensive care unit to facilitate the initial post-operative healing. In surgeries that involve extreme pain or cause a shock to the body's system—like separating conjoined twins—this prolonged sedation helps patients get through the tough early part by keeping them still and comfortable. This type of anesthesia creates a state like suspended animation for patients, slowing them down and maintaining them in a controlled environment.

As for the rhythm of their work, anesthesiologists are like firemen. They're either sitting around the firehouse and playing cards or running off to a fire. Typically, they're hanging back because the patient is doing fine with the medication used. The heart is beating, blood pressure stable, breathing regular. They're bored because they did such a good job that nothing goes wrong. There's no in-between: There's either a fire or they're playing cards. Frankly, with my anesthesia, I'd want them to play cards. But if I have a problem, I want to be sure that they know how to put out a fire. Remember, you're asleep. You can't exactly plead or discuss your options with them.

Anesthesiologists have been trained to think clearly and act effectively in an emergency. Time and again, I've been amazed at how coolly and professionally these unsung heroes react.

Here's a snapshot of the medical equivalent of a four-alarm fire:

It was like something out of a movie. All I did was turn my head, and instantaneously there were seven additional anesthesiologists in the room. They simply materialized, seemingly out of nowhere.

The child on the operating table had gone into laryngeal spasm, which is one of an anesthesiologist's worst nightmares. At the beginning of any surgery requiring general anesthesia, the anesthesiologist puts a tube down the patient's throat. This gives the doctor more control over the patient's breathing. The real trick, though, is getting the tube out (extubation). This is a critical time in anesthesia. For obvious reasons, with a tube shoved into it, the larynx, or voice box, can become very irritated. And it's not necessarily a function of how long the surgery takes. It can happen during short cases as well as long ones.

When the anesthesiologist pulls the tube out, the larynx can clamp down, cutting off the oxygen supply. Having a cold or other upper respiratory illness increases the chances of laryngeal spasm. This is why surgery is often postponed if the patient has a cold; the risk is too great. When the larynx closes, you have only a few minutes to reopen the airway before the patient can get brain damage from a lack of oxygen.

Anesthesiologists use a few quick techniques to alleviate a laryngeal spasm. The anesthesiologist tried them all but still couldn't open the airway. So he pushed an alert button, and within seconds, what seemed like an army of anesthesiologists appeared. I heard nothing, but our group went from three people to nearly a dozen in a flash.

Working together, the anesthesiologists were able to reopen the airway in a matter of seconds. They gave the boy large doses of muscle relaxants to halt the spasm, then threaded a very thin tube—about the size of those little cocktail straws you get in mixed drinks—down his throat to deliver oxygen. Once that was in place, they were able to insert a larger tube. This they left in until after the child woke up.

It's important to understand that the original anesthesiologist did nothing wrong. He responded correctly to an unforeseen problem. People assume that when a problem occurs in the operating room, it's the result of some blunder. In my view, most problems occur because something unexpected happened and people don't know how to respond to it. Fortunately, here they did.

Anesthesiologists do sometimes have to make life-and-death decisions in a split second. You can think of it as defensive driving. They stay alert and maneuver so as to avoid collisions. That's the kind of driver I want at the wheel.

LEVELS OF ANESTHESIA

The American Society of Anesthesiology groups anesthesia into four basic levels:

1. Minimal (a medication like valium, which takes the edge off pain)
2. Moderate (conscious sedation)
3. Deep (analgesia)
4. General

Up until general anesthesia, the patient should be breathing on his own. Under general and sometimes deep anesthesia, the patient is breathing through a tube controlled by the anesthesiologist. Within each category, there are varying levels of anesthesia.

You can ask what level of anesthesia you are getting and why that level is most appropriate for you.

A note on outpatient surgery. Much surgery today is done on an outpatient basis. The impression is that it's not a big deal. But when it's surgery done on you, it is a big deal. Within the American Society of Anesthesiologists, there is discussion as to whether an anesthesiologist is needed for moderate sedation. In nonhospital surgical centers, people other than anesthesiologists are administering anesthesia more and more frequently. My personal opinion is that this is not okay, and that people are being misled to think that sedation is a minor matter. It isn't.

Once my daughter was going to have surgery that involved general anesthesia. The choice was whether to have it in the doctor's office operating room, or in the hospital. I requested the hos-

WHO ADMINISTERS ANESTHESIA?

Anesthesiologist (M.D.). This is the gold standard: a medical doctor who has completed four years of college, four years of medical school, and a four-year anesthesiology residency program in a hospital. They then take the American Board of Anesthesiology examination and become board-certified. Some go on to fellowships in an anesthesia subspecialty for another year. Anesthesiologists provide or participate in more than 90 percent of the estimated 40 million anesthetics administered in the U.S. each year.

Certified Registered Nurse Anesthetist (C.R.N.A.). This is a registered nurse who has completed an extra two years of specialized training in anesthesiology.

Surgeon (M.D.). In some plastic surgery centers, your surgeon may be the one administering anesthesia. You want to know this before you agree to the procedure.

My personal opinion is that it's too much to be responsible for the patient's heart rate, breathing, and consciousness if you're also performing surgery. If the doctor's just removing a mole on the arm, that's one thing. But if the patient is going to be sedated, as in deep sedation, there should be another medical professional, such as a nurse anesthetist, in the room.

Anesthesiologist's Assistant-Certified (A.A.-C.). Commonly known as an anesthetist, this person has passed a national certification exam upon completing an accredited anesthesiologist's assistant education program. Find out if the supervisor, an M.D. anesthesiologist, will be present at all times. If not, ask how many rooms the supervisor is covering. I would say that any more than two rooms is too many.

Registered Nurse (RN). Depending on the requirements of a given state's Board of Nursing, registered nurses are allowed to administer intravenous drugs under your doctor's supervision and to monitor your vital signs.

pital. The doctor's nice secretary told me how wonderful they were there. But I was thinking that I didn't want to be in a position to find out if she knew CPR; I wanted the OR nurses, who have seen every kind of situation. Mild sedation—on the level of valium or some similar drug—is one thing, but any time general anesthesia is required, you need to be particularly vigilant.

SERIOUS BUSINESS

Most people facing surgery are primarily concerned about the qualifications of their surgeons. As well they should be. But few give so much as a thought to the anesthesiologist or nurse anesthetist who, quite literally, holds their life in his or her hands while they are unconscious during surgery.

The fact is, even if—God forbid—it goes wrong, most surgery isn't going to kill you. Sure, there are some exceptions. Putting something in, you can put it in wrong. Taking something out, you might not take it all out. And rearranging things, you can muck them up. But unless you're dealing with the blood supply to the head, heart, or lungs, you're probably not going to kill the patient. That doesn't mean the patient will be happy with the results if something goes awry; I'm not saying that. The point is that the patient is unlikely to die. If surgery doesn't come out right, you may be able to get it fixed or redone (that's called a "re-op"). With an anesthesiologist's work, if it doesn't come out right, you're done. That's it.

The surgeon can do a masterful job on your surgery, but if the anesthesiologist doesn't respond correctly and you have a complication on the operating table, that is not a good thing. And if the anesthesiologist doesn't work well as a team with the surgeon during a complicated operation, you're not going to get the same result as if they have worked out a rhythm together.

This in no way takes away from the skill and judgment of surgeons, because they have to react quickly to the unexpected as

THROUGH A SURGEON'S EYES

This happened just as I was writing this chapter: A thirteen-year-old girl named Madeleine is having eye surgery. Everything is going fine. Anesthesiologists who work with eye surgeons know to look for an ocular/cardiac reflex: when an eye muscle gets pulled, the heart rate may drop. I pulled on the second eye muscle and the anesthesiologist stopped me—the heart rate had gone *up*. This was very peculiar—it usually decreases. It went from 100 to 169, and then went back down to 100. "Now you can proceed," she said. I then alerted her: "Now I'm going to pull on a muscle." Nothing happened, and so we went on with the surgery.

Toward the end of the procedure, a new anesthesiologist, Dr. Anthony Clapcich, came on; this because of the rules about anesthesiologists' hours. When he took the tube out, the girl's heart rate went up and stayed high. In the recovery room, Dr. Clapcich called in one of the pediatric cardiologists to evaluate. At this point, the parents were getting worried. Everything had seemed fine, and now two doctors and a battalion of nurses are coming in, along with a defibrillator. The cardiologist gave her a medication—adenosine—and the girl's heart went back to a normal pace. They were able to break the attack.

There are arrhythmias that develop during puberty. Here, the anesthesia "uncovered" it. Madeleine was able to go home after surgery without problems. However, she needed to come back for a full cardiac work-up.

Again, this was unusual, unexpected, and taken care of appropriately. A successful effort to avoid problems doesn't mean that there are no problems; it means that you've been able to avoid worse problems. The parents were quite upset. Their daughter was fine walking in, and now she was seen to have cardiac problems. They found it hard to understand that sometimes things happen. The surgery with anesthesia uncovered a problem that no one knew about before. The final diagnosis was Wolff-Parkinson-White syndrome, a specific variety of arrhythmia. The anesthesia, an abnormal situation, probably triggered the expression of this existing arrhythmia.

well. But it's important to understand what a crucial role the anesthesiologist plays.

IT TAKES TWO

When you arrange to have surgery, you're actually picking two doctors: You're choosing the surgeon, and the surgeon's institution is choosing the anesthesiologist.

Anesthesiologists are highly skilled medical doctors. In addition to assisting the surgeon during surgery, they anesthetize patients during certain medical tests (such as angiograms, MRIs, and certain radiological tests) and administer medication to manage pain (morphine, Demerol, or lesser pain medicines). Their role has expanded in recent years with advances in the medications and technology in the field.

Under general anesthesia, you are asleep. You are totally dependent on the anesthesiologist to keep your blood pressure constant and your vital signs strong. The best anesthesiologists understand the surgery the surgeon is performing as well as the physiology involved. During certain kinds of surgery, the patient's blood pressure may go up and down. If the patient's blood pressure goes too high, there's blood all over the field and the surgeon can't see, or you blow out a blood vessel. If the blood pressure drops too low, the patient can have a stroke on the operating table. A good anesthesiologist knows how to anticipate this.

In the pediatric operating room at Children's Hospital of New York, there has *never* been an anesthetic death. We deal with children with severe cardiac problems, children who receive heart transplants, children with serious neurological problems, rare muscle diseases, you name it. We have nine operating rooms that have been busy with surgery five or more days a week over several decades. This is an extraordinary record, and we aim to hold it.

I treat a lot of very sick children, some with serious neurological problems. In cases involving serious medical problems (such as children who have had previous cardiac surgeries or those with certain genetic syndromes, such as Down's syndrome), I order what is called an anesthesia consult. I do this not the morning of the operation but well before so that the anesthesiologist can go over the child's medical history and discuss any special tests they might want done. We may bring in relevant consultants, like the patient's cardiologist or pulmonologist. We go over the essentials: What will the surgeon do? How long will it take? What kind of anesthesia is needed? How will the patient's disease modify the anesthesia?

We try to tackle all the problems we can in advance. For example, we may pretreat the patient with medications in order to steer clear of a potential complication. As a team, we come up with a plan for how this child will be put to sleep so that we can do what we have to do.

The anesthesiologist will then talk to the child's parents. Has the patient ever had problems under anesthesia? If the child did have a problem at another institution, they would get the chart and find out what drugs were used so as not to use the same ones. Or they would plan to use that drug in combination with another medication that will eliminate the problem. There are numerous ways to accomplish the same thing. The anesthesiologist's tool kit contains preparations for analgesia (pain relief) and for inducing amnesia (forgetting). In certain instances, they might do more of one than the other.

Several chapters ago, we met a CEO who underwent surgery in a community hospital and suffered a serious complication—his esophagus was cut. When he came to New York for a re-op, he was surprised that the anesthesiologist wanted to look at EKGs and his entire medical record. "He's only doing my neck," he said. "What does he want to know all this stuff for?" That's the point: The anesthesiologist was being thorough in his job. He wanted all this information so that he could avoid potential problems during the surgery.

THE IMPORTANCE OF TEAMWORK

A good question to ask your surgeon is, "How often have you worked with the anesthesiologist who will be putting me to sleep?" If they haven't worked together much, ask your surgeon if there's an anesthesiologist he or she *has* worked with a lot, and whether that person is available for your surgery.

The surgeon and anesthesiologist have a close working relationship, as if performing a duet. You need people who can read each other, guessing each other's moves in advance. If I tell the person I'm working with, "Please keep the patient deeper for a little while," he'll know what I mean because he's done the procedure with me before. When I say, "Five more minutes," he'll know what my five minutes mean. This is why many surgeons only want to do surgery with certain anesthesiologists. The more complicated the procedure, the more this comes into play.

Before I begin surgery on a child, the anesthesiologist will ask whether it's okay to use a certain anesthetic agent. And I will say yes or no. They ask me because the drug they're considering may affect parts of the body also affected by the surgery. In my case, as an ophthalmologist, that means the eye muscles. In other instances, it may affect blood pressure, muscle tone, or heart rate.

The anesthesiologist will also ask me for an estimate of how long the surgery should take. And I'll give him one. This is significant because some medications in their repertoire are shorter-acting, and some are longer-acting. The anesthesiologist then drugs the patient accordingly.

Toward the end of surgery, I'll give the anesthesiologist a warning bell. If my warning bell is consistent to the minute, he can titrate the medication exactly. He will have begun to reverse the anesthesia so that the patient regains consciousness at the optimal time. The goal is to use the smallest level of anesthesia mediation necessary. This is particularly true of a child—because of size—and someone who is ill. If the anesthesiologist is not familiar with children, or has not been exact, the patient can wind up being sedated for too long. The patient might lie there sleeping for another half hour or more after the surgery is completed. It's not a terrible thing, but someone who is oversedated will feel groggy and generally out of it longer than he should. If you have two people who can talk to each other and are used to each other, it goes a long way.

SPECIAL EXPERTISE

Doctors who administer anesthesia fall into specialty categories. To be a specialist within anesthesiology, the doctor will have had at least one additional year of training, passed a qualifying test, and had his credentials evaluated by the governing subspecialty body—all of this only after they have completed basic anesthesiology training and been certified by the American Board of Anesthesiology. The subspecialties within anesthesiology are pediatric anesthesiology, neuro-anesthesiology, cardiothoracic anesthesiology, and pain management. They may all look the same to you, but each has special areas of expertise.

Many smaller places have certain specialists, such as a pain management specialist, but a larger hospital would have most specialty areas represented. This doesn't necessarily mean you're going to get the specialist. If your basically healthy child is to undergo what is considered routine surgery, the pediatric anesthesiologist is more likely to be tending to the seriously ill children with airway problems, where his expertise is paramount. You may need to actually make the request. How you do this— and how successful you will be—depends on the place. However, it can't hurt to make a polite request. They can always say no.

I'm not saying that an adult anesthesiologist can't work on a child; nor would I say that an adult ophthalmologist can't examine a child. But there is a difference. A pediatrician is going to do a different exam on a child than an internist would. Given a choice, you would rather have the pediatrician—whose frame of reference is children's health—examining your child. And given a choice, you would ideally or at least frequently have an anesthesiologist who works with children all the time administering to your child. With children, the doses and range of acceptable medications in anesthesiology are different from adults. Unless you're in a major medical center, children's hospital, or sophisticated suburban hospital, you will probably have a general anesthesiologist doing adults and children. And that's fine, as long as they do a lot of children.

Similarly, if you're having a procedure where a particular subspecialist would be most appropriate, you can put in a request. If not, make the point that you would like to have the anesthesiologist that your surgeon is used to working with.

At the very minimum, you are entitled to know the certification level of the person administering anesthesiology to you or your family member. Ideally, this is a board-certified anesthesiologist. But often this is a nurse anesthetist. At the Harkness Eye Institute of Columbia, for example, we have one anesthesiologist supervising nurse anesthetists. The nurse anesthetists perform low-level sedation for routine, uncomplicated cases. But there is always the ever-present anesthesiologist for back-up and ongoing commentary. And if he thinks that a case warrants his involvement, he steps in.

The combination of experience and specialization is crucial in surgical anesthesia. When planning surgery, you want to make sure that the anesthesiologist has a good deal of experience with the type of surgery you're about to have and is experienced with the patient population you represent.

Yes, you can ask.

SUSPICION SAVES A LIFE

Before any pediatric surgery, one of the things we check is whether there is any family history of malignant hyperthermia, a rare but extremely serious muscle reaction to anesthesia.

This is what happens: An enzyme secreted by the muscles triggers a rapid rise in heart rate. In turn, the child's temperature goes through the roof—up to 105 degrees or so—and he can suffer cardiac problems. This is dangerous and potentially fatal.

It happens very quickly. In the early stage, the heart rate goes up more than expected in response to one of the anesthetic agents. In one case, the anesthesiologist had just started the anesthesia when he asked me to cancel the surgery. The evidence wasn't clear, but he suspected malignant hyperthermia. The signs for this are rapid heart rate, irregular heart beat (arrhythmia), and a rise in temperature. However, the symptoms don't always arrive in a neat package. He said, "I think this is what's going on, but I'm not sure. And I don't want to find out." I said, "Fine. We can schedule this again."

He couldn't quite articulate what it was that bothered him. In some circumstances, the heart rate can rise without there being a problem. But his index of suspicion was high enough to yell stop, even though he knew what a big deal it was to cancel an operation once it had begun. And I never overrule an anesthesiologist.

It turns out he was right. The reaction shows up in enzyme levels, much as will happen in a heart attack patient. We kept the child in the hospital, monitoring him closely, and twelve hours later the blood we had taken at the time of the anesthesia verified that he had malignant hyperthermia. Because malignant hyperthermia worsens over time, subsequent blood levels were even higher. He saved the child's life. But even if he hadn't been right and the child didn't have malignant hyperthermia, he still was right to follow his instincts. That's how you eliminate problems.

In the future, any anesthesia request for the child will have a warning attached to it. But because this anesthesiologist caught the early warning signs, no damage was done to the child.

HOW DEEP IS THE POOL?

In certain places you can request your anesthesiologists, while in others you can't. In general, in the smaller private hospitals, you can. In the bigger places, you might not be able to, or there might be limited choices within the area of specialty.

In some places, you will have a nurse anesthetist or a nurse anesthetist with an anesthesiologist supervising. There are several different arrangements. It generally depends on the institution and what surgery is planned. For example, some hospitals have anesthesiologists on hand for childbirth; others don't. In the ones that don't, sometimes a mother who needs an epidural block or emergency cesarean-section has to wait for an anesthesiologist to be brought in. If you're about to undergo a procedure that might require anesthesia—as in childbirth, where the need for anesthesia isn't predictable—you should know whether an anesthesiologist will be present.

I once saw a case where the anesthesiologist's presence during childbirth proved critical:

Everything in the operating room seemed in order. It was Barbara's first pregnancy, and she was having twins. During an office visit close to her due date, the obstetrician, an excellent doctor named Edward Bowe, M.D., said that it was time to do a C-section. He finished with his patients, then personally walked her over to the delivery room for the operation. Within moments, twin boys were born healthy and fine. One of the boys had the cord around his neck—twice. Because the babies had been delivered quickly by C-section, there were no problems. Had there been a problem, the neonatal intensive care specialists from across the hall would have arrived in force like a SWAT team. But had Barbara gone into labor, that one child might not have made it. Also, it turned out that Barbara had placenta previa, which meant that the placenta had been covering the cervix; this condition can be fatal to the mother during labor. Why did Bowe decide to do a C-section? His only explanation was, "Something bothered me." (Are you starting to see a pattern here?) Score one for our hero. And score one, too, for Barbara and her husband for deferring to a fine doctor's judgment.

After the C-section, for no apparent reason, she started hemorrhaging severely. Dr. Bowe and the anesthesiologist were starting to get nervous. They gave her blood via transfusion and stopped the bleeding. Dr. Bowe left, then came back a few moments later. (Something "bothered" him.) She was hemmorrhaging again, losing large amounts of blood. She had Disseminated Intravascular Coagulopathy (DIC), which means that the clotting mechanism turned on itself, causing intensive bleeding. They continued to transfuse her and ultimately stopped the bleeding. All told, she lost fully half of her blood volume. The entire time, the anesthesiologist controlled her blood pressure, kept her sedated, and performed complicated vascular tricks with his medication to keep her from hemorrhaging more. Thanks are also due to the nurse who quickly responded to the problem and stayed on top of the situation.

There was a particularly poignant episode of the TV show *ER* where the same thing happened. A healthy, young pregnant woman gave birth and then started bleeding profusely. She died in the delivery room. Her newborn was left motherless. That's what would have happened here had it not been for the fast thinking and skill of the anesthesiologist, the surgeon, and the nurse.

Barbara was an otherwise healthy woman who just happened to get the bad luck of the draw; these were completely random, unexpected complications. When Dr. Bowe told me this story, he was literally shaking, so unnerving had this been—decades of obstetrical experience notwithstanding. But this was an extremely rare occurrence, a rare occurrence that happened to a healthy person. Bad things do happen to good people, as Rabbi-turned-author Harold Kushner put it in his best-selling book. The best defense is to know that the backup is there if you need it. You can pick a hospital that has a team of highly skilled medical professionals ready to respond instantly if something bad does happen.

Since you don't usually get to vote on which anesthesiologist is assigned to your surgery, you may as well pick the place that picks the best anesthesiologists. Which means a high-caliber medical institution. The important thing is not whether you can request your anesthesiologist; rather, you want to know that whoever puts you to sleep for your surgery is chosen from a deep pool of highly skilled anesthesiologists.

If you want to make sure, you can get the name of the anesthesiologist slated for your surgery and check with the hospital to see whether the person is board-certified in anesthesiology. Your surgeon should be able to answer these questions. You can also learn whether the anesthesiologist has a subspecialty certificate or is recognized by the American Society of Anesthesiologists as a subspecialist in an area related to your surgery. If a nurse anesthetist is assigned to your surgery, you can make sure a board-certified anesthesiologist will supervise.

Note that sometimes the anesthesiologist isn't assigned until the day before the surgery, or even that morning. This is the result of the ever-changing dynamic of the doctors' on-call schedule and laws governing how much they can work. At our hospital, they will usually assign the same anesthesiologist to a patient who has had previous surgery with us, and will at least try to honor specific requests.

CHAPTER EIGHT

The Radiologist

T HE FIRST DAY OF OUR INTRODUCTION to Radiology course in medical school, our professor showed us an X-ray. We knew it was the chest because we could see the ribs and the clear lungs.

"What does this X-ray show?" the professor asked us. There were 120 eager-beavers in the class, all very smart, all of whom would go on to become physicians. And every one of us looked blankly at the X-ray, completely baffled. We saw before us two U-shaped shadows. Not one of us had a clue as to what those mysterious shapes were. We might as well have been trying to decipher ancient Egyptian hieroglyphics.

"Those," the professor finally informed us, "are breasts."

We all laughed. It was really very funny. I mean, this was a fully mature woman and there was really nothing ambiguous about it. You couldn't have missed it!

But we did.

The episode taught us an important lesson: An X-ray is only as good as the person reading it. Technically speaking, it may be faultless. The picture may be sharp with clear contrasts, in perfect focus, and without a hint of movement on the part of the patient. But if the person reading the film doesn't know what he or she is looking for, it's worthless. To the uninitiated eye, these were just lines on an X-ray. None of us would ever mistake breasts on an X-ray again.

That's why a radiologist is so valuable. Radiologists are among the hospital's key detectives. They're looking for visual clues, things most people wouldn't even notice, to put together into patterns of diseases. First, you have to know how the disease looks. You don't read an X-ray in a void. People who interpret these tests need to have knowledge about the diseases that affect the area in question. Even though they don't actually treat the disease, they have to know about the disease and the different ways the disease appears. In other words, they have to know what's potentially there in order to see it. Otherwise, they may trip over it. A radiologist has to have a sense of the range of what's normal or abnormal in a given situation. Sometimes it's not so clear which is which, and the radiologist will need to exercise judgment.

Reading X-ray film is not like reading the words on a page. Most abnormalities don't leap off the film at you. They can be extremely subtle. One disease may look like this. Some exceptions within that disease category may look like that. If the radiologist doesn't know the variations, he might assign the wrong diagnosis.

We rely on radiologists to read highly sophisticated visual tests and then draw the appropriate conclusion about what's wrong. We count on them to know where in the haystack to look for the proverbial needle. So much hinges on how well they do their jobs.

A good radiologist is worth his weight in gold. If you build a house on an insecure foundation, everything that follows will be skewed. In the same way, radiology provides the foundation for the diagnosis of certain conditions and diseases. If you don't have the right diagnosis, or you have a slightly wrong diagnosis, or the severity is misjudged, then your treatment plan is based on an incorrect foundation.

For example, if a tumor shows up clearly on a mammogram, that's one thing. You have to take a biopsy. But if you have a shadow from a calcium deposit, or fibrocystic disease (a benign condition marked by lumpy breasts), it can be very confusing. Your radiologist might order an ultrasound to try to sort out these differences. If there is any doubt as to whether it's a tumor, a calcium deposit, or a cyst, you might still have to have a biopsy because you don't want to take chances.

This is where a top-notch radiology team comes in. If they can finesse the details on the X-ray, it can save you a biopsy. Let's say that a biopsy is needed. If the surgeon does the biopsy and misses the piece, then you think you don't have anything abnormal. That happens. So they'd better perform the biopsy on the right spot. Sometimes the surgeon needs target guidance—which radiological tools can provide.

A friend of mine, Caroline, had a mass show up on her mammogram. She found an excellent surgeon, one with whom she felt comfortable. The surgeon had another radiologist mark the spot with a needle. Then, when the surgeon went to take the biopsy, she followed the tip of the needle to the mass. The radiologist (1) found the mass on the mammogram; and (2) gave the surgeon a laser-guided missile with which to locate the spot to biopsy. The sample would then go to the pathologist, who would interpret the cells.

The two radiologists—one who read the mammogram and one who provided the guidance—and the pathologist were integral to the process of determining whether the mass was benign (open the champagne) or not. If the mass were found to be cancerous, three other doctors would step forward: The pathologist, internist, and oncologist would help determine the stage of disease, the radiation oncologist would assist if radiation was needed, and the oncologist would supervise any chemotherapy. And all these physicians came with the package once Caroline picked her surgeon. While you can seek opinions on your own from oncology and radiation specialists, you most often stay within the orbit of the doctor you have chosen.

You also need the test to be done correctly. And that's where the assistants, or techs, are invaluable. Just as a surgeon does a dance with the OR nurses, the radiologists do a dance with their assistants. If the X-ray isn't taken correctly, it won't be read correctly, which means that the diagnosis won't be right. It's simple: If you don't get the correct information, you can't make the conclusion correctly.

A great deal goes into getting an X-ray done correctly. The patient has to be positioned just right. Doing it once instead of four times—to limit the time, discomfort, and radiation exposure—certainly helps. And so does looking at the right area.

RADIOLOGY SUBSPECIALISTS

The subspecialties within radiology are pediatric radiology; interventional radiology; neuroradiology; and radiation/oncology. Within these specialties, the radiologist may play a role in treatment as well as diagnosis. Radiology used to be just broken bones and chest X-rays. In the last fifty years, the radiologists' purview has broadened considerably.

PEDIATRIC RADIOLOGISTS

Pediatric radiology is self-explanatory: Pediatric radiologists have expertise diagnosing disease in children. There are many diseases unique to children. And because their bones are still developing, reading children's X-rays is quite different and difficult. Pediatric radiologists also seek to limit radiation exposure for children. For example, when CAT scans are done on children, doses are decreased by a factor of three. This is particularly significant in children with chronic diseases, as with the girl with the ovarian cyst, whose condition will be monitored by radiation-based tests.

In general, only large urban medical centers have pediatric radiologists. If a child has an unusual or complicated series of tests, the results should be read or reread by a pediatric radiologist because adult radiologists are not as familiar with children's diseases and their manifestations.

VASCULAR AND INTERVENTIONAL RADIOLOGISTS

Vascular and interventional radiologists use sophisticated radiological tools for various treatments. This is a relatively new area. Interventional radiologists use dyes, microwires, and catheters, which allow them to isolate abnormal blood vessels or blockages and identify abnormal webs and patterns. For example, they can thread extremely tiny tubes into the blood vessels and then inject a dye. The pattern in which the dye lights up helps them diagnose disease.

A fine example of this is the heart angiogram. An interventional radiologist threads small tubes up through the venous system from the patient's groin. When he gets to the point where the vessels feed blood to the heart muscle, he will inject a dye and take pictures to see what happens to the dye. He know the appearance of normal patterns. If there's coronary artery disease, the blood vessels will be very narrow in certain areas and thus the pattern of the dye will be thinner than in healthy vessels. If there's a blockage, the tree branch will end. The radiologist reading this will see that the heart is pulsing and the blood in the vessel has hit a dead end. On the basis of this information, the surgeon will make treatment decisions.

Interventional radiologists can also use the same pathway to treat and cure. For example, some children have what's called an atrial septal defect (ASD), a hole between two chambers of the heart. Today, a vascular and interventional radiologist can thread a special device through the vessels into the heart to close the window between the two chambers. Fixing these so-called "holes in the heart" used to require major, open-heart surgery. Only when there are extremely large holes is this the case now.

Mr. Smith's surgery—to treat the vascular malformation behind his eyes—was a similar treatment in a different physcial area. Indeed, these tools can be used in many parts of the body. Here, the interventional radiologist put the guide wire in far enough to reach the exact spot. The dye was then inserted so that the problem, a vascular web, was identified in detail. That was the diagnostic phase. The treatment phase involved threading baby wires into the web of vessels. Each wire was "turned on" and the abnormal vessels were burned—and thus shut down. This was done on each branch of the web. It took hours. But it was done perfectly by a master radiologist, one of the few in the country who could have done it.

When my father was found to have a mass in his abdomen (the enlarged lymph node), and it needed to be assessed, a radiologist assisted in the biopsy. Rather than cutting him open to get at the mass, the radiologist, using ultrasound, provided a laser-guided target. Using a needle, the urologist treating him took a small sample to be read by the staff pathologists. This was similar to the way Caroline's surgeon relied on radiological tools to guide her biopsy.

Amniocentesis, a procedure used to diagnose fetal defects, is much the same thing: The ultrasound helps the doctor find the precise spot to sample. Today, most obstetricians perform their own amnios with ultrasound guidance, and then a pathologist evaluates the cells.

NEURORADIOLOGISTS

Neuroradiologists do head and spine CAT (computerized axial tomography) scans, MRIs (magnetic resonance imaging), PET (positron emission tomography) scans, and other sophisticated scans of the head and spinal cord with very specific variations. Neurological diseases are different, and require a high level of expertise.

When Mr. Smith's doctors were working toward a diagnosis, he had several CAT scans of his head. The first was a head CAT scan, which was normal. When the first neuro-ophthalmologist was looking for a specific type of tumor that was not fully isolated on the first scan, he sent Smith back for another series. Later, the diagnosis had shifted, and Dr. Behrens thought there was a vascular web behind the eyes. He had our neuroradiologist reread the first two CAT scans. The neuroradiologist didn't see the area that Dr. Behrens wanted to look at, so Dr. Behrens ordered a third CAT scan from a neuroradiologist to look carefully at the area behind the eyes. This scan was consistent with a vascular web (bruit) behind the eyes, but also with thyroid eye disease, which was not high on the list of possible diagnoses. So he requested a further test, an angiogram by an interventional radiologist, to provide the definitive answer. If the web were identified, the diagnosis would be made. And Mr. Smith could be treated at the same time. This is exactly what happened.

RADIATION ONCOLOGISTS

Radiation, directed by radiation oncologists, is integral to cancer treatment. Many complicated decisions go into which radiation protocol a patient will be put on. For example, the total dose may be a certain number of rads. But the details are significant: How many doses? How often? Over how long a period of time? What exact area of the body will be treated?

Radiology is a field of great precision. A couple of millimeters one way or the other makes a huge difference. The treating radiologist will determine how the patient is to be positioned, as well as the machine settings, and the technician will carry out these instructions under the physician's supervision. On subsequent occasions, a technician will follow the script and the radiologist will give approval. Once the technician has correctly positioned the patient and focused the machine, a cast may be made so that the patient doesn't move. The technician will put the patient into a cast and mark his or her body. (The marks look like blue or black Magic Marker, and they have square edges.) Basically, this is the outline of the beam to be used. The table doesn't move. The machine is at a set distance, and the grid on the patient's abdomen ensures that the window pane is going to be a certain size. The edges of that grid are marked so that when the patient lies down on the same table, with the machine in the same place, the beam is projected onto his or her belly with the precision of a laser pointer. Once the positioning is complete, the tech will hit the pedal.

When the radiologist and techs are very precise and, indeed, neurotic about lining you up, you're going to get more precise treatment. Is it a bad thing to not have the more precise treatment? I don't want to be the one to find out. In the better places, with the better doctors getting the better results, they don't just get the better results by themselves. They get the better results because the people around them are excellent *and* they are closely supervised.

There are new variations on the classic radiation treatments. Patients will often receive small doses in small, targeted areas. For example, with prostate cancer a radiologist may insert radiation seeds directly into the prostate to kill off just the prostate cancer cells and a small amount of surrounding tissue. It's like a time-release capsule, and the radiologist establishes the dose, how long it lasts, and how far it spreads. Cervical cancer patients may get radiation through a tampon of sorts. In certain eye tumors, a plaque, a flat object resembling a coin, is sewn against the eyeball and removed once the treatment is complete. In all of these cases, only the tumor itself and a small area around it receive the radiation.

PARTNERS IN DIAGNOSIS

A very good doctor will read his own scans. But each doctor will have favorite radiologists to work with. As always, it goes back to communication and responsiveness. An internist or other specialist may say, "John, I'm looking for X in a patient. When you do the scan, look for this particular manifestation of the problem." For example, Dr. Behrens reread the CT scans on Mr. Smith with our neuroradiologists. When he was looking for the "web" behind the eyes and needed another scan, he told the neuroradiologist exactly what he was looking for and the neuroradiologist knew exactly how to find it.

With, say a chest X-ray to rule out pneumonia, it's usually pretty straightforward. But depending on what the physician is looking for, the radiologist may add cuts. "Cuts" are individual views. You can think of it like cutting a loaf of bread. You can cut it several ways: into four pieces, into eight pieces, or you can take one chunk and divide it into several skinny pieces. If a Cracker Jack ring is stuck in the loaf of bread, you'll have to cut narrower slices in order to find it. Radiologists can't do narrow cuts on everything; they have to choose what to focus on quite carefully.

CT scans and MRIs are pictures taken different ways; CT scans involve radiation and MRIs do not. Also, CT scans are better on bony areas; MRIs on soft tissue. In either case, the radiologist takes a series of photos. In a general head CT scan, a certain number of photos, spaced a predetermined way, are taken. When Dr. Behrens was hunting down the web, the area behind the eye was targeted. The space intervals were tiny; he didn't want to miss anything by skipping an area. It was like a manhunt in a two-block area, apartment by apartment, as opposed to a manhunt citywide.

CHAPTER NINE

The Pathologist

WHEN I WAS STUDYING at the Washington University Medical Center in St. Louis, a woman in her seventies came in for treatment. She was from a farm in nearby Iowa. Based on her blood work, her local doctor had concluded that she had a fatal type of leukemia and had referred her to our hospital. She believed, and we all believed, that she had a bad disease and a terrible prognosis.

This was a job for pathology. This woman had been sick for a long time and clearly did have something wrong with her. But when our pathologists reviewed her blood work, they discovered that, in fact, she had a benign blood disease that only *resembled* leukemia. The doctors at the rural hospital had treated her very well, but they were perplexed by what she had. Nobody mistreated her; nobody made a mistake. This was an extremely complicated case that required high-level detective work. It took a group of high-level pathologists an entire week to figure it out, but upon very careful comparisons of slides, they determined that her illness was not fatal.

This woman was like everyone's grandma, always smiling, always trying to make *us* feel better, even though she was the one supposedly dying of a terminal disease. She was just a fabulous woman. And I had the privilege of saying to her, "They made the wrong diagnosis. You're fine. And we can fix your problem." The other physicians allowed me to be the one to tell her because I had developed a relationship with her. This was really a kind of favor to me. It was the first time I was ever able to say something like that. It was thrilling.

And I have never had the privilege of being able to do this again.

Among physicians, pathology is considered one of the most intellectual and scholarly specialties, for its practitioners need to have a working familiarity with the entire range of diseases. At the same time, people outside the field know very little about what pathologists actually do. Other physicians, to say nothing of the general public, often lack the vocabulary with which to talk about the pathologist's work.

WHAT PATHOLOGISTS DO

A pathologist looks at tissue samples and establishes the presence or absence of disease, or analyzes the results of tests on blood, urine, cerebral spinal fluid, or other body fluids. If there is disease, the pathologist will determine which subgroup it falls into. The pathologist is the arbiter of disease patterns. If, for example, your internist or surgeon suspects cancer, everything usually hinges on the pathologist's report. Data from the pathology department represent the single largest number of transactions in a patient's medical records; it's estimated that 70 percent of all hospital information systems is devoted to pathology. Yet despite the crucial and pervasive nature of their task, pathologists remain largely invisible to the public.

Ralph Green, M.D., Chairman of Pathology at the University of California, Davis, tells a joke that conveys a sense of the pathologist's place in medicine:

"An internist, a psychiatrist, a surgeon, and a pathologist went duck hunting. A duck flew overhead. The internist took out his binoculars and said: "I think it is a mallard but its markings aren't quite right." He took out his Audubon guide and flipped through the pages. By the time he found the illustration, the bird was gone. The psychiatrist saw the next duck, raised his gun and took aim. He stopped and mused: "This could be an endangered species of duck. If I shoot this duck then I will be conflicted. If I don't shoot it I will be hungry. Hunger will cause me to become introspective. What shall I do?" The duck disappeared, out of sight. As soon as the next duck flew by, the surgeon raised his gun and fired. The bird dropped out of the sky. The surgeon turned to the pathologist: "Go get it and tell me what it was!"

As surgeons, we're used to people making fun of us. In my profession's defense, however, I would say that the pathologist in the story wouldn't have had the duck to look at had the surgeon not gone out and caught it! Medical specialty jokes—collegial but slightly competitive—are part of our world. They keep things light. But like all good humor, there's a bit of truth within the bite.

To be honest, before embarking on this chapter I didn't even know where the pathologists at our hospital worked. I knew it was a great department, but otherwise it was a complete mystery—a black box. Pathologists do much of their job in their laboratory, often set apart from the bustle of hospital life, and few others give much thought to what they're doing. But their conclusions may well be pivotal to the very physicians who know so little about their actual work.

PATHOLOGY'S ROLE IN MEDICINE

Pathology is the study of the nature and cause of disease. It is a rarefied field, calling upon arcane knowledge and detailed laboratory expertise. Think microscopes and slides, only we're talking very high-tech, high-resolution microscopes and slides that have undergone elaborate preparations and tests.

Many people associate pathologists with autopsies, and rightly so. But that's only a small part of what most pathologists do. Pathologists are part of every medical evaluation of a patient's blood or tissue. Any time some tissue or a tumor is removed from a patient, a pathologist examines it. This is the law.

In operations I perform, I may remove eye muscle or pieces of eye muscle and/or surrounding tissue. I send it to pathology. Afterwards, I receive a memo that states: "This is normal tissue." Were I to have a case with abnormal pathology (i.e., tissue found to contain abnormal cells), I would have some interaction with those in the pathology department who deal with muscle tissue. Given my specialty, this would probably involve neuropathology or pediatric pathology. But so far this has not happened, and pathology has remained an abstraction housed in the nether reaches of the hospital.

Columbia-Presbyterian has thirty-five board-certified pathologists on staff. According to Charles Marboe, M.D., the chairman of Columbia-Presbyterian's pathology department, in order to cover the specialties relevant to patient care, a medical institution should have at least five pathologists: hematology (blood); neuropathology; cytopathology (cellular pathology); pediatric pathology; and dermapathology.

At larger hospitals, the pathologists subspecialize and see slides only from patients in narrow areas, such as (1) general surgery; (2) tumors; (3) cardiac; (4) ob/gyn; (5) hematology/oncology (which includes lymph tissue, bone marrow, and solid tissue); (6) bone; and (7) liver. It's a lot like the police force: In a small town you may have five policemen who do everything. In a big city, however, you'll have crowd control pros, expert marks-men, and personnel trained to handle hostage situations. They will have specialists in areas we don't even know exist. But we're glad they're there when the need arises.

When I write that a pathologist will "see slides" in a particu-lar area, understand that the slides are the pathologist's "patients"; pathologists interact with medical patients via the slides that hold their laboratory samples. A pathologist sees patients from the inside out. They work from the particulars as revealed through the slide and rarely come in contact with the actual patient. By con-trast, an internist will deal with the whole person, and then address particular problems as the need arises. It's a different ori-entation. Among the specialties within pathology, hematologists or the pathologist who runs the laboratories that process speci-mens are the most likely to interact with patients. Pathologists also run blood banks and assess patient reactions to blood transfu-sions. Another group that may deal directly with patients is the cytopathologists, who perform fine-needle aspirations for biopsy purposes. While surgeons and oncologists often do fine-needle aspirations, the procedure was developed within the field of pathology.

BIOPSIES

Pathologists evaluate biopsies. Biopsy literally means "observa-tion of the living." A sample—a piece of tissue or part of an

HEMATOLOGY

Hematology is the branch of pathology that deals with the red and white blood cells. There are many different subgroups. Hematologists have expertise in blood-related diseases, specifically leukemia and lymphoma. Immunohematologists (called immunopathologists) also do blood typing, tissue typing, and the measurements of cells and blood compatibility for transplants.

organ—is taken from a patient for observation and evaluation. A sample of fluid, such as from a cyst or other body cavity, can also be examined. While a surgeon or other specialist usually does the actual specimen removal, the pathologist is responsible for observing and evaluating that specimen. The pathologist looks at the sample under a microscope to see if the cells are normal, cancerous, or precancerous. Because of increased breast cancer awareness, many people are familiar with breast biopsies. They are the most common. After that, the most common biopsies are prostate and then, due to more frequent colonoscopies, gastrointestinal (GI). A lung biopsy would take place in the hospital; breast or prostate biopsies might be done in the hospital or in a physician's office. If the doctor wants to examine fluid in a breast cyst, for example, a needle biopsy performed in the physician's office would be the most likely approach.

When a physician takes a piece out of somebody, it is immediately put into a fixative solution, such as formaldehyde, to preserve it. The solution used is determined by the type of tissue. The sample is then embedded in wax in the pathology lab. Then, ultra-thin slivers are shaved off for examination. (This is done much the way meat is cut in the deli.) The slivers are put on a microscope slide and stained with different chemicals to bring out different parts of the cells. Depending on what the pathologist is looking for, in accordance with the disease in question, he or she will examine different pieces. The main chunk—the source of the slides—should remain intact. This is important to know: You should always be able to get additional slides for another opinion.

In the case of Sarah, the young girl with the ovarian tumor, her parents brought the original slides to expert consultants. They went to two fine institutions for additional opinions and met with a pediatric oncologist and pediatric surgeon in both places. Each had a pathology subspecialist read the slides. Everyone agreed with the diagnosis that she had a specific subtype of ovarian tumor. Had they not agreed, this would have changed the course of events, and the biopsy would have been evaluated further. Their analysis of the tumor determined the treatment: The pathologist and the surgeon at one of the hospitals were on the cutting edge of research and treatment in this area, and according to the latest statistics, patients with this exact type of tumor seemed to do fine with neither surgery nor chemotherapy. On the basis of the pathology report, the parents decided to have their daughter followed rather than undergo aggressive treatment. Five years from now, this girl will be part of the group that will have made her treatment the mainstay for this subtype of ovarian tumor.

STAGING WITH PATHOLOGY

You may recall that one of the physicians who saw Sarah had recommended a laparotomy to "stage" the cancer—to see how advanced and extensive the cancer was. A pathologist would have been instrumental in the process. In a staging laparotomy, the surgeon biopsies the abdominal organs and takes samples from each cluster of lymph nodes in the abdominal cavity. Then fluid is put in the abdominal cavity and the doctor does what's called "washing," taking samples of the fluid as it brushes against the affected area in the abdominal cavity. It's a bit like taking a swab of your mouth. The exact approach will vary depending on the suspected disease. For example, ovarian tumors might spread in a different way from pancreatic ones. The pathologist takes a set volume of the fluid and spins it so that the heavier tissue cells fall to the bottom and can be removed for further analysis. The pathologist will identify the cancerous and noncancerous cells and assess the cells in question to establish their subtype.

The biopsies read by pathologists were also central to my father's course of treatment for prostate cancer. He had a mass in his abdomen, which the surgeon was going to treat as if it were metastatic prostate cancer. However, I had been taught that you find out what you have before you operate on it. My father switched doctors. The new urologist and radiologist said that with this particular combination of test results, they would have been surprised if this turned out to be cancer. But they checked.

PROSTATE BIOPSIES

With prostate biopsies, the pathology department gives every prostate cancer sample what is called a "Gleason score." This is a rating of severity on a scale of 1 to 10, with ten being the most severe. The prostate itself is about the size of a chestnut. In a prostate biopsy, a little piece will be taken from several different areas. This is because the tumor is not spread out evenly; in one spot, the cancer may be severe while in another spot, it may be mild or nonexistent. Pathologists have a procedure to reconcile these variations, which ultimately yields a composite score. Based on the score, your doctor will design your treatment.

But a score of five may be read as a four or a six depending on the institution. The score chosen will have ramifications for treatment and prognosis. The treating physician will rely on judgment, in combination with the clinical examination and laboratory tests. Pathology provides one significant layer to the foundation for making key decisions. With my father, they determined that, based on recent research they had done together, the Gleason score did not suggest metastatic cancer.

That was one part of the pathology evaluation. The second was to answer the question: What was this thing in his belly? He had a needle biopsy—with a radiologist-guided fine needle—done under anesthesia. A sample was taken from the mass in question, which the pathology department then read. Had the pathologist deemed the sample cancerous, he would have established the variety and my father would have been treated accordingly. The pathologist saw normal lymph tissue, merely part of an enlarged lymph node. The pathologist made the final conclusion, which changed my father's treatment.

As we've discussed, proper surgery, or really any form of treatment, comes only after correct diagnosis. What the pathologists do is nail down the specifics. Yet they do this behind the scenes, so patients usually don't know about them.

Pathologists work on the level of subtle distinctions and variations. When they inspect a sample, the diagnosis rarely jumps out fully formulated. To evaluate a sample, they observe it under the microscope using complicated stains to see how the cells appear. The manner and extent to which the cells bind or do not bind to certain markers will help them assess the patient's health. For instance, the pathologist may put dyes or antibodies, which would have been prepared in the laboratory to bind specifically to the slide sample, on the different pieces. He or she will watch to see if, say, dyes number one and two bind but not dye number three. This will tell the pathologist something about the patient's condition.

The work of the pathologist requires the same kind of thought process as does diagnosis. The pathologist begins with a hypothesis, tests that hypothesis, and then confirms the hypothesis. He or she draws on extensive knowledge of the patterns and presentations of different disease states. The pathologist understands conditions that are both common and obscure and knows when to suspect which one.

I can't emphasize this enough: These pathologists determine your fate. In the sense that their conclusions about your disease will determine what treatment you receive, they are like the three Fates of Greek mythology, whose job it is to spin the thread of a person's destiny. You will never know their names, you won't see them, and you may never know they exist. But they are the ones who make the difference.

FROZEN SECTIONS

Biopsies are often performed on the spot during surgery. During the operation, the surgeon takes what is called a "frozen section." After the surgeon takes a biopsy or excises a tumor, the tissue is brought to the pathologist. It is frozen so that he or she can cut a piece from it (hence the term "frozen section"). The pathologist slices it and puts a sliver of it on the microscope.

This happens right in the operating suite. The pathologist has a little booth off to the side, which is equipped with a microscope and the ability to do first-round stains; fixing the tissue and embedding it in paraffin would take time, and the surgeon needs the pathology report to know how extensive the surgery will be. The pathologist takes the sample and stains it to determine the specific subtype of cells it contains. This determines the subcategory of disease, which by extension will help determine the patient's treatment. This can be done for any tissue in the body. For instance, a biopsy may be done to determine whether a mass on the lung detected on an X-ray is benign or malignant. And if it is malignant (cancerous), the pathologist will identify the category of the tumor. The answer is not always immediately evident. There are premalignant tumors, with cells that aren't quite normal but have yet to cross over the threshold of disease. How such borderline samples are assessed depends on the pathologist's judgment.

The pathologist's findings often determine the remainder of the surgery. When excising a cancer, the surgeon wants to be sure that he has removed all of it. A cancerous tumor will have boundaries, but there's generally some seepage. The surgeon sees where the tumor appears to end, but will know that cancerous cells may spill past the line. As a result, the surgeon will take out a little more than the seeming boundary would indicate—a margin. The margin that needs to be taken for particular tumors has been established through years of study. Sometimes the surgeon will think that it has all been taken out, but then needs to go back and remove a little more. Rather than wake up the patient and do it again, the patient will remain under anesthesia until the pathologist ascertains when the correct margins have been reached.

In a staging operation for cancer, the pathologist's task is to determine how extensively the cancer has spread, something that cannot be established until the patient is asleep and in surgery. Take, for example, a radical prostatectomy (abdominal removal of the prostate for prostate cancer). The surgeon will take a biopsy of the lymph nodes near the prostate, which the pathologist will examine to see if the cancer has spread to the lymph nodes. If not, the lymph nodes are left alone. If the cancer has spread, the operation will continue and more tissue is removed.

In many large medical centers, pathologists are assigned, on a rotating basis, the job of being on-the-scene in the OR. Whoever is sitting in the hot seat is making some pretty hefty decisions. If the on-site pathologist finds that he can't make the ruling, or if there's someone else with expertise in the area of tissue removed (heart, lungs, etc.), he will immediately page the expert. The expert pathologist will then drop everything and *run* to the OR (because everyone recognizes that the patient is under anesthesia and thus time is of the essence) for consultation. Frozen sections are very important because the surgeon wants to be certain to get the proper disease status and take the proper margins. A pathologist has to have a certain warrior mentality. He has to make a recommendation based on extremely fine distinctions, and all the while the surgeon is breathing down his neck. It's fine when the situation is clear-cut. But there are those gray areas when judgment prevails. The surgeon wants to do right by the patient. The pathologist wants to do right by the patient and the surgeon. It's important to recognize that the pathologist at the surgeon's side is making his recommendation based on information available at that moment—that's where the pressure comes in.

There is an interaction between a surgeon and a pathologist. The pathologist is focusing on the details on the cellular level, the knowledge of which informs the surgeon's work. In the meantime, the surgeon's broader knowledge about the patient can help the pathologist put his findings into context. The surgeon may say, "This patient is a smoker," or, "This patient works in a coal mine," or "I am taking biopsy from an area which has been operated on previously." The pathologist may then think, "Oh, that explains why those cells are reactive—this is scar tissue." The surgeon can relay information specific to the patient that helps the pathologist read the signs. This is why their ability to communicate is important. They're detectives on the same case, but each has a different beat.

At the same time, the tests that pathologists select and conduct will determine how a surgeon or other physician sees a patient's condition. On any given case, they can't do every test known to science but rather must choose efficiently. They know what do to get the information they need. Knowing where to look is as important as anything else, and a good pathologist will know.

AUTOPSIES

Another of the pathologist's responsibilities is performing autopsies—examining a dead person to better understand the cause of death. We think of this as a gruesome, unpleasant task. Granted, it's hardly glamorous. But this is how we know about the course of so many diseases. Historically, bodies were not allowed to be studied. The first brave individuals who wanted to see how we were put together had to resort to grave robbing in order to study the body.

The very first course you take in medical school, an extensive one-year course with lectures and labs, is anatomy. The laboratory part involves the dissection of a human being. The knowledge of anatomy you derive from this provides the basis for everything else you do in medicine. When the time came to meet our dissection subjects, we were all terrified. This was no longer like taking college classes with tougher tests. This was the real deal. We had an extremely kind professor, a premier anatomist named Dr. Peterson, who was used to taking rookies through this medical school rite of passage.

I will never forget the day when my medical school group walked to the back of the room to find 25 steel beds. We were walking into a field of dead people, and it was very strange. Every person was lying face down, their defining features obscured. We were all dumbstruck and fearful of what we had to do, but we knew we had to do it. This was more than a matter of being handed a cadaver to work with. This was crossing an invisible portal: Our lives as regular people lay behind us; our lives as doctors lay ahead. We felt the wonder and awe of being led into the inner sanctum, where only a few—fellow doctors—have been before. This was a quiet but transformative event. This was our coming of age.

Dr. Peterson clearly understood what a profound experience this was for us and talked us through it gently. He told us how these people very specifically gave their bodies so that we could learn and become physicians. Frequently, these people had sent letters to medical students describing who they were and wishing them a good career. It was clear that they had taken pride in knowing that they had participated in the making of a physician. We treated our very first "patients" with great respect.

When a patient dies and the treating physician believes that an autopsy will shed light on the circumstances of the person's death, he or she will request permission from the next of kin and order an autopsy from the pathology department. Our hospital has an autopsy rate of 10 percent. About 6 to 7 percent of adults who die will be autopsied; the number is higher for children. There are different sets of rules and regulations as to how you do an autopsy, depending on whether the patient has died from unnatural causes, such as a head trauma or a knife wound in the abdomen, or from an underlying known or suspected disease. The autopsy will be organized based on the pathologist's hypothesis. Also, states have different laws regarding who performs autopsies. In some states, the medical examiner is not required to be a pathologist.

The popular CBS show *CSI: Crime Scene Investigation* is all about pathology. There's a crime, and the medical examiner's office strives to figure out how the person died and to find the culprit. In one episode, somebody noticed ridges on the victim's fingernails. They knew that lead and certain other poisons leach out through the fingernails. This helped them figure out that the person had died of heavy metal poisoning and identify the exact metal. Pathologists often work backward, figuring things out by observing changes in certain organs and running chemical tests. *CSI* also shows the kind of high-end detective work pathologists do with DNA and special stains that respond to specific wavelengths of light. This is Sherlock Holmes at its best.

CREDENTIALS

To be an accredited pathologist, someone must go through four years of medical school, complete a year of internship, and do a residency in pathology for four years. A pathologist will then take the American Board of Pathology written examination, a very rigorous test with a substantial failure rate. This is an exam for each of the nine specialties. Becoming an expert in a pathology subspecialty requires additional years of training, and yet another exam.

Many specialties within pathology require additional testing. The following are a mere sampling: blood banking/transfusion medicine; chemical pathology; cytopathology (working on the level of the individual cell); forensic (applying medical knowledge to matters of law); hematology (blood); medical microbiology; neuropathology; and pediatric pathology. Pathologists may also work in conjunction with skin specialists (through the American Board of Dermatology) as dermatopathologists, and in the field of molecular genetic pathology, through the American Board of Genetics. These people have often done two residencies and taken board-qualifying exams in two areas. At this time, however, there are no specific tests for general surgery, cardiology, ob/gyn, and tumor pathology subspecialties.

Pathology is a highly regulated field. Not only are there firmly established rules for how individuals' tests are done, but laboratories must continually undergo proficiency tests and subscribe to proficiency programs in order to remain accredited. Beyond this, all laboratories are regularly inspected by the College of American Pathologists in the most minute detail. To give you a sense of how seriously this is taken, the inspectors pore through the procedure manuals (some two thousand pages each) for every test the lab carries out and check the log that records the refrigerator temperature. Sound nitpicky? If the refrigerator is faulty, the reagents for the stains could deteriorate. The number of factors to be monitored in the pathology lab is mind boggling. No other part of the hospital has such regulation.

HOW YOU CAN TAKE CHARGE

To minimize any chance of a mix-up with laboratory tests, you can physically take your test and walk it to the lab. If you're not able to walk your sample down yourself, you can ask a nurse to do it for you. Some hospitals will view this as intrusive and others won't. But you can always ask.

When you go to a hospital, the staff pathologists come with the deal. So the best way to ensure that good pathologists are on the case is to pick a good hospital or medical center that's large enough to accommodate a fair range of specialties within pathology.

If you are at a smaller hospital and would like a subspecialist in pathology to evaluate your tests, or if you would like a second opinion, you can arrange this quite easily. For a fee, you can send your laboratory slides to a pathologist anywhere in the country. Breast cancer patients are beginning to take advantage of this. But for the most part, very few people do this or even know that it's an option.

This is what you do: At the time of the test, ask for extra slides to be made. The pathology department at your hospital will put the slides in a special box. Then call the pathology department of a renowned medical center—try the chairman of pathology's office directly—and say, "I would like my slides reread." They will ask a few questions and direct your slides to the appropriate subspecialist.

Many insurance companies will reimburse for the reevaluation of slides. The fees run from about $150 and up, depending on how extensive the testing. But trust me—this is not a big money-maker. This is a service. And the highly expert pathologist you consult will be part of your care. If you're dealing with a complex problem, the pathologist at your home hospital may suggest mailing a sample for a consult. Whether it's on your own or your doctor's initiative, however, the expert's observations can be considered. If the pathologist's conclusions contradict or add specificity to your diagnosis, your physician will talk to the pathologist, and together they can assemble a plan of action.

This is the way it should work. But sometimes egos get in the way. Your doctor or the staff pathologist may say, "Don't you trust me?" As soon as you hear that, there's only one thing to do: switch doctors. The smartest doctors say, "Fine. Get more opinions. I'll help." It's the nervous, insecure ones who say, "Don't."

If your lab results come back and you are told that it's something serious, you should get a second pathology opinion. If you start off with something that appears simple and you get back an uncertain pathology report, get a second pathology opinion. It's easier to do through your own doctor, but with a little homework you can figure out where to send it.

Let's say you have an unusual or complicated problem and you want to pursue a second opinion, or perhaps even a third. You want to locate the person who's an expert in your area of concern, the pathology guru of the subspecialty. You can:

1. Call the American Board of Pathology [(813) 286-2444], and ask who the leading specialists are in the area of your diagnosis. Now go to step number three.

2. Or, call a fine medical center and ask for the pathology department. Ask what subspecialties they have represented to find out if yours is among them. If you have a cardiac problem, and they don't have an expert in your area, locate the hospital that does. It's fine if a generalist does the first round. But as a medical consumer, you should know that there are subtleties that a subspecialist would be more prone to grasp, and that you have access to such subspecialists.

3. Ask how to send the slides for consultation. You need to know the address; the mode of transport (hand delivery, regular mail, Federal Express, etc.); what paperwork needs to be done; fees; and any medical history they will want to have from you.

Remember, you're just shipping your slides around. You're not shipping *yourself* around. And these tests may mean everything, folks.

CHAPTER TEN

Nurses

―――――∿―――――

I N THE DAY-TO-DAY, MINUTE-BY-MINUTE life of the hospital, the nurses are everything. When you have a problem post-surgery and need a painkiller, the nurse will tend to you. When you're waking up from an anesthetic, the doctors may be in and out of the room, but the nurses are hovering over you. The physicians diagnose, make treatment decisions, and perform surgery; they oversee the patient's medical care. But the ones who implement care on the most immediate, hands-on level are the nurses.

Nurses are the ones who assess a person's comfort relative to his or her condition—and can do something about it immediately, because they're there. That's the crux of the matter. If a change in the patient's condition warrants attention, they bring it to the supervising doctor's attention—because they're in the room and see it first.

If you have a cast on and your leg starts to swell, they'll notice it at the earliest phase. If you're becoming less communicative instead of more—which may be the first sign of a reaction to a medication or a post-surgical complication—they'll pick up the subtle cues. It's easier to fix small problems than it is to fix big problems. This is why nurses are indispensable.

Like other medical professionals, nurses develop areas of expertise. There are several nursing specialty areas, some of which require additional training or certification. The type of work nurses do may also evolve through inclination and experience. The categories I describe are: (1) Floor nurses (RNs); (2) Intensive Care Unit (ICU) nurses; (3) Operating Room (OR) nurses; (4) Labor and Delivery nurses; and (5) Trauma Center/ Emergency Room nurses.

FLOOR NURSES

When people think of nurses, the first to come to mind are floor nurses, those who may care for patients over a period of days or even weeks. The stereotype is the nice lady with the white hat, tucking patients in their beds and dispensing warmth and cheer. This picture greatly underestimates nurses' expertise. It is also inaccurate: You're unlikely to see a Registered Nurse (RN) changing sheets today. Tasks requiring little medical expertise are now delegated to Licensed Practical Nurses (LPNs) and Nurses' Aides, while RNs have been nudged up into more supervisory roles. This has created tension within the system. The ranks of nurses have been stretched thinner, and fewer numbers of RNs are being given more responsibility.

People want nurses to be saintly. But it's hard to be saintly when, as a group, you're understaffed and are therefore forced to set priorities. For like everyone else in medicine today, nurses are

CREDENTIALS

To qualify as a registered nurse (RN), a candidate must (1) graduate from an accredited nursing program; and (2) pass a rigorous national exam. Some states have a continuing education requirement. For more information, visit the American Nurses Association at www.nursingworld.org.

running faster to do more. As a professional group, nurses are very upset about this. They feel great dedication to their patients and lament any organizational changes that interfere with good care.

As a medical consumer, you must recognize the climate within which today's nurses function. This way you can pick your battles in your quest to secure optimal care—which is what I needed to do when my husband was recovering after back surgery. For the entire day immediately after the operation, the nurse practically lived in the room. The close attention he received was appropriate; this was just after the surgery and, accordingly, the nurse assigned to him was given fewer patients to take care of. The evening of the following day—this was a different shift—Len needed a shot of the narcotic for pain before he went to bed. I was visiting him at the time, and he was getting quite uncomfortable. He made the request at 11:00. I went home at 11:15. My mistake was going home before he got it.

Len asked for the medication again at 11:30. At that point, I talked to him and found out that he still hadn't received the medicine. I called the floor nurse at 11:40. "Yes, doctor," she said. Then I heard from Len, "Still no pain medication." So at 11:47, I called the nurse supervisor for the floor unit and said, "Give him a shot." I knew how the hierarchy worked, and he got his medicine. But it had taken almost a full hour. Part of the problem was that he had only asked for it when he was uncomfortable; like many patients, he had been trying to keep his pain medication to a minimum. By the time he got the medication, he was upset and in pain. Mind you, he was not in any danger, but his level of discomfort was unnecessary and inappropriate.

When I showed up the next morning in uniform—wearing my white physician's coat—the nurses on the floor were nervous. They were afraid I would complain.

I didn't. Here's why: First, I didn't want anyone to take it out on Len; and second, I knew that nursing departments are understaffed, even in the best places. An institution will try to stretch the staff on the floor rather than in the OR or ICU. The hospital is not going to cut in areas where a nurse's presence is a question of life and death. If they trim staff, and patients get angry or frustrated, that's another matter. Also, I knew that RNs are the only ones who can give a patient a narcotic. Narcotic dispension is very carefully regulated. Two nurses are required to open the narcotics box and sign out the specific medication and specific dose. Freeing up two nurses on one floor can be difficult, so Len didn't get his medication for an hour.

Also, I would make sure that this didn't happen again. I knew that Len was about to be discharged. Mentally, I made a cost-benefit analysis: It wasn't worth making more of a fuss because this was a short-term situation.

Everybody who has been to the hospital has a story like this. With all due respect to professionals, nursing shortages in hospitals make such situations more common. This doesn't make it right, but it is the reality we're all confronting. The strategic response is to be vigilant and make sure you or your loved ones receive proper attention, without stepping on anyone's toes.

ICU AND CCU NURSES

The nurses who work in the intensive care unit (ICU) or cardiac intensive care unit (CCU) are goddess-like figures. They work in a narrow field and are extremely quick to respond in critical situations. In particular, they become highly adept at recognizing problems among high-risk patients who may change course rapidly. They develop a deep understanding of the norms in a given setting so that any time a patient's response deviates from that norm they will pick up on it. They are monitoring the blood pressure, checking that the IV is dripping sufficiently, and ensuring that the patient is breathing well with the particular respiratory settings.

The ICU nurses are executing orders from the doctor. If we compare the goings-on of a hospital to a military operation, ICU nurses would be the infantry. They execute orders from the doctor and react deftly to changes. If a patient vomits, the nurse makes sure that he is cleaned up and that the medication went down. Much of what they do is also organizational. They check on procedures and keep the doctor apprised of the patient's condition. If they note anything of concern, they can bring it to the doctor's attention. They serve as a screening system for the doctors; they are the first line of defense.

In the neonatal ICU, where premature infants and other newborns are closely watched, one nurse will be responsible for two babies. By comparison, two physicians might be responsible for overseeing the entire unit. The nurses are working on a micro level, watching patient changes in real time.

The observational skills of the ICU nurses are everything. While they don't have the medical doctors' expertise, they become familiar with the specific problems that crop up among specific groups of patients. They know what's normal and abnormal in the diseases they tend to. For instance, a nurse who works with neurological patients will know the appropriate level of alertness following one type of surgery as opposed to another. He or she will know that a patient who has abdominal surgery faces different complications than a neurosurgery patient. The nurses know how problems differ depending on the surgery and the patient group. For instance, pediatric and adult patients face different respiratory risks post-surgery. The ICU nurse will also know how to work with the assigned population. To give one example, nurses in the neonatal ICU become masterful at inserting IV tubes into tiny patients.

As in the rest of medicine, a large part of observation is knowing what you're looking for. A really smart nurse who makes the effort can become extremely knowledgeable about the class of disease she deals with. For instance, the woman who runs the pediatric ICU at Columbia-Presbyterian knows more about how her patients respond to treatment than do some of the newer baby doctors who pass through. This is because she is continually observing and treating this group of patients and has been privy to problems that a physician may come upon merely once or twice during a career. She and the pediatricians have specific fields of knowledge, which complement each other.

This is more than simply cooperation between nurses and doctors; it's an interaction between people whose expertise and responsibilities overlap. There's redundancy in what each knows, and that redundancy protects the patient. The physician addresses the patient and the disease from a medical perspective. The nurse tends to the person who has the disease and the problems that arise with the disease.

When something happens, ICU nurses can react immediately. If a problem surfaces outside their realm of responsibility, they bring it to someone's attention. Different medical institutions may assign ICU nurses different levels of responsibilities. This generally depends on the degree of disease in their patients, and whether the hospital has residents. As with the doctors, there's a very distinct hierarchy among the nurses as a group, with senior nurses being in charge.

Nursing floors generally run on three eight-hour shift rotations. In the ICU, however, the day is divided into two twelve-hour shifts. With critically ill patients, it simply takes too long to get a sense of how to take care of the person. If the shifts are shorter, by the time one has a feel for it, another shift starts. The longer time frame allows the nurse to be truly expert in a given patient's condition and needs.

OR NURSES

A good operating room nurse knows the operation at hand. She might not be qualified to perform it, but she will know the nuts and bolts of the procedure as well as the idiosyncrasies of the surgeon. From a surgeon's point of view, this makes the work go faster and more smoothly. You're not waiting around for some-body to find just the right suture because the suture is already there. And if once in every ten times you use a different suture, that one's there too—because the nurse has anticipated this.

This isn't just knowing how an operation proceeds when it goes well, but knowing what to do when it doesn't. It's like danc-ing. Take Ginger Rogers and Fred Astaire; he led but she followed him in sync. A good nurse will know what's happening, *and* know how to anticipate problems and how to fix them, *and* know what a given doctor will want in the way of tools and approach.

At our hospital, the OR nurses have a series of index cards that they use to keep track of different operations. For example, the card will note that, for this operation, I like to use a specific suture with a specific needle. Before the operation starts, the nurse will go over the card. Then he or she will ask me, "Do you need something special today?" I may say, "Yes, this is a re-op. I will need more sutures, or a steroid-antibiotic injection to prevent scarring." This may not have been obvious from the information available to the nurse beforehand.

I have my beloved OR nurse, Arlene, whom I could not live without. When Arlene does an operation with me, I don't even look up anymore. I just take the instrument she hands me because she knows what comes next. When Arlene is on vacation or out sick and I have a substitute, I spend a lot of time making sure the tray has all the instruments I need before the case. During the pro-cedure, I may spend significant time looking on the tray for one instrument or another because he or she doesn't know what to give me. If the instrument isn't there, the nurse may have to go to the storage area around the corner and wait for it to be sterilized if it hasn't been already. This is not because the nurse isn't well trained or competent, but because he or she isn't accustomed to working with me. It's all part of the ebb and flow of surgery. With Arlene, my ability to proceed from one phase of surgery to another without stopping to ask a question or check on my tools makes the whole thing go more easily. Having a substitute nurse in the OR with me doesn't put the patient at any greater risk; it's just not as smooth.

A subgroup of OR nurses work in the recovery room. The recovery room is, in effect, a type of ICU with the nurses arrayed in much the same way. They are very much on top of the patients' needs and they develop a similar expertise with post-operative patients. Similarly, they are assigned few patients, generally two. With many operations, including neurosurgery and open heart surgery, the patient's immediate status may be determined by medication. The moment the patient is emerging from the anesthetic is crucial. Whether the patient is woken up or sedated again will be critical to the healing process. The micro-management of this process is done by nurses.

In the case of the young girl who suffered an arrhythmia during eye surgery, the OR nurse was continually at her side. Two nurses had the defibrillator prepared, should she need her heart rate converted. If this had proved necessary, one nurse would have assisted the doctor and the other might have been with the parents, keeping them calm and reassured through this unforeseen event.

The recovery room nurses react immediately to changes in the patient's condition. They know what to do for the kinds of things that happen: a blood vessel pops; a patient's pain exceeds the normal range; an EKG reading suddenly changes and suggests a problem. They know when to bring in the anesthesiologist. At any given time the doctors who care for the patient are not far away, but nurses are at the patient's side.

LABOR AND DELIVERY NURSES

The delivery room nurse may be watching the fetal monitor while the obstetrician is darting in and out of the room. The nurse will alert the doctor to any problem he or she doesn't see. If labor is being induced, a nurse absolutely must be in the room at all times. And in all labors, a nurse must be present after a certain point. She might go out for a few seconds, but will be just outside the door. The patient is not alone during labor. It is important to have that assurance. The nurse will notice something happening and bring it to the attention of the doctor, who might have walked away for a moment, or call in an obstetrician, who hasn't yet arrived.

When Judy delivered her baby, the delivery room nurse needed a push. Which fortunately, her husband, Tony, was able to provide. As she recalls, there was a real run on the maternity ward that day; it was two days after Mother's Day *and* the full moon. Whatever the reason, the beds were full and Judy was tucked into a small closet-like room off the main wing.

Tony noticed that the fetal heartbeats displayed on the monitor seemed to be slow. He knew that the fetal heart beats faster than an adult's heart, so a slow heartbeat might be a problem. He pressed the buzzer and the nurse who had set them up, clearly harried, came in. She seemed to have already decided that since this was a first labor, it was going to be a long but uneventful (yawn) process. Any perceived problems would no doubt be due to the parents' anxiety. "Sometimes the machines aren't hooked up right," she said. "That is probably what happened here." She jiggled the wires, checked that the fetal heartbeat was normal, and left the room.

Tony saw the heartbeat slow down again and worried: This was not the machine. He pressed the buzzer again, and a different nurse came in. This one reacted quickly. In less than a minute, Judy was moved to a larger, better-equipped room and—out of nowhere, it seemed—her doctor, flanked by an entire surgical team, stood ready to do a cesarean. She was given an oxygen mask to breathe through so that the baby would have sufficient oxygen. She dilated quickly, so Brendan was born without the drama of surgery. The cord had been wrapped around his neck; hence the varied heartbeat. It was nerve-wracking, but everything turned out fine.

The initial nurse's reaction made Tony question his instincts. But he had enough confidence in his perceptions to call the nurse again. It's important to know that in such instances, you don't have to be right. You can simply have concern or doubt and want things to be checked. You can say, "I may be an anxious parent, but.... " You can be firm but polite.

In some hospitals, a licensed midwife, supervised by a doctor, will tend to patients. Other places won't have midwives, but the delivery room nurses will have a great deal of autonomy. Once again, a nurse can bring a fetal arrhythmia to the doctor's immediate attention. Ultimately, this may lead to an emergency cesarean to assure the baby's well-being. This happens all the time.

I am very indebted to the delivery room nurses who tended my labors. They helped me immensely with the huffing and puffing part. When I got anxious, they calmed me down. They were able to create a calm setting during an inherently anxious time. This made things better for me, better for my husband, and better for the baby. When the doctor arrived, I was reassured to know that I had been in good hands. Referring to the nurse, the doctor had said, "You got a good one."

TRAUMA CENTER/ EMERGENCY ROOM NURSES

Other subspecialty nurses work in the emergency rooms or trauma centers. Nursing specialty areas include: surgery, emergency, pediatric, psychiatric, and nurse-midwives. Many specialties have their own organization and credentialing, and many require additional study or certification.

As a group, the subspecialty nurses here are usually among the best and the brightest in the profession. Why? They're doing complicated tasks in a fast-moving arena. These are not leisurely settings. The nurses that specialize in critical areas are both self-selected—they have to want to do this intense work—and selected through the process. The nurse needs to hand the correct instruments to the surgeon who needs it *now-now-now*. The concept "in a little while" does not exist. They need to be absolutely on top of things, even able to anticipate what may happen next.

THE NURSE-PATIENT RELATIONSHIP

Nurses can interact intimately with families. They can respond to comfort issues, such as if the patient is too hot or too cold. They see what's happening and may be able to give family members a broader, more inclusive description of what the patient is experiencing than the doctor.

Because they devote more intensive time and have more body contact with patients, they can be soothing. They can be a source of reassurance and encouragement. Indeed, they are trained to interact with people in a comforting way. Also, as they are not at the top of the hospital's power pyramid, many patients and patients' families find nurses more approachable. Sometimes a physician will ask a nurse to pose a question to the patient, not as a means of passing the buck but so that it's more comfortable for the patient. For example, when a doctor wants an answer to a question that he doesn't think the patient will answer directly, he may ask the nurse to ferret it out—knowing that the patient may find the nurse less threatening or judgmental.

Everyone thinks they're going to go to a great hospital to get a great doctor, but what you really want is a great team. You need a team where the doctor, the assistant, and the assistant's assistants work together efficiently and reliably to ensure your comfort and safety. As the Harvard Business School study showed, it's not the surgeon's expertise alone that guarantees a good outcome; it's often the doctors' and nurses' abilities to work as a team.

SENIORITY AMONG NURSES

Nurses know the seniority within their group. By this I don't mean chronological seniority—who has been there longest—but rather intellectual and experiential seniority. And they'll often assign the most challenging or sickest patients to the most competent nurse. For instance, in the neonatal ICU they might assign a baby who's clearly thriving to a nurse relatively new to the setting. The most difficult cases will be dealt to the most senior nurse, not to the rookie. This is done very quietly and you can't control it. Everything gets prioritized according to the patient's level of need.

Here's a case that demonstrates how nurses are instrumental in a patient's care:

You may recall that Jenny, my friend's sister, was to undergo a stem cell transplant as a treatment for multiple myeloma, a type of blood cancer. She had found an internist who could act as an intermediary with a top specialist in the field and keep tabs on her treatment. Well, even the most thought-through plans don't always pan out. The internist got sick. Since the stem cell treatment leaves patients extremely vulnerable to infection, the internist wasn't allowed into Jenny's secured room. The family was devastated.

Enter one fabulous nurse practitioner. She saved the day. She was in charge of a few patients, and she didn't miss a beat. The transplant went as smoothly as such a complicated procedure possibly can.

It's not that you don't get problems; it's what you do when you get them. People assume that a lack of problems means nothing went wrong. Really, what happens with good care is that someone puts out the brush fires so you don't get forest fires. In medicine, you don't just do something; you do steps one through ten in a given procedure. If you notice a problem at step two, you can more easily change course than if you notice it at step five.

It's like a high-wire act: If you make it to the end of the rope without falling, it's not necessarily that you didn't almost fall, but that you caught yourself so that you didn't fall. This nurse practitioner was so in command of things that, procedurally, everything went right. If anything had gone wrong, she would have caught it.

There's a lot of back and forth between doctors and nurses. Stereotypically, this has meant the arrogant doctor ordering around the well-intentioned nurses. But this dynamic has, thankfully, been put behind us. Frankly, any doctor who treats nurses disrespectfully is foolish because so much in medicine depends on what nurses do.

The nurse functions as an additional layer of observation between the doctor and the patient, another person paying attention to what's happening to the patient in the here and now and acting as the patient's advocate. A nurse may remark to a physician, "I think this patient is having such-and-such a problem." And that may prompt the doctor to reevaluate the treatment. It's not a matter of "us" (the doctors) and "them" (the nurses). It's all of us.

AN EVOLVING PROFESSION

Nursing has become a well-paying profession—and it commands the respect it deserves. However, the ranks of trained nurses have thinned. One reason is that many women who, in previous generations, would have become nurses are now going to medical school. Another is that many nurses are employed outside the hospital as high-level technicians or assistants to doctors. For example, in many surgical offices, a staff nurse serves in a sense as the doctor's alter ego. She is the gatekeeper; all questions go to her. Such nurses may have a great deal of knowledge about a set of problems and procedures. With my husband's back surgery, for instance, I had no question that the surgeon's nurse couldn't answer. If there had been one, she would have asked the doctor and then conveyed his response to me.

In many medical practices of all types, nurse practitioners may see patients under a physician's supervision. Other physicians may refer patients to nurses for information on ongoing problems or upcoming procedures. Nurses also perform administrative roles, such as screening claims at HMOs. Others hold key positions in, or even run, medicine-related organizations.

In some medical settings, nurse anesthetists administer many types of medications. While they are supervised, they're still making decisions on an ongoing basis and carry a great deal of responsibility. Many places will assign a nurse anesthetist instead of an M.D. anesthesiologist to a case. The question, of course, is which do you want in a given situation. (As seen in Chapter Seven, The Anesthesiologist.)

Today, an increasing number of men joining the nursing profession are filling in the gap. Often these are medical professionals from other countries who, because of difficulties with language or the limits of their training, can't get other higher-level jobs. The stringent qualifications in this country make it very difficult to transfer as a physician. In New York, for example, many male nurses come from the Philippines, Ireland, and Russia. Also, women are rediscovering nursing as a profession that offers flexible hours—appealing in this era of two-career family life—and the chance to really make a difference in people's health and well-being.

GETTING THE BEST CARE FROM THE NURSING STAFF

While you can choose your own doctor and even request your anesthesiologist, you can't request your nurse. That's a fact. You simply get the person who's been assigned. But there are two things you can do: (1) have a family member there to ensure that you get proper, timely care (see Chapter Eleven, The Patient's Advocate); and (2) pay for private duty nurses. However, once

THE GIFT

Every year I buy ten cases of Girl Scout cookies and give them to the people I work with at the hospital. I started doing this when my eldest daughter was a Girl Scout, so she could get the stuffed bear— the prize for the biggest seller. Now it is my annual way of saying thanks.

As I was walking to the operating room one day, I realized that the thing people don't understand is that it's not me. When an operation is successful and a child's sight is saved, it's not due to any magic on my part alone. It's that there are all these people I work with who do their jobs and help make me look good.

My mother had recently been in the hospital for eye surgery. Let me tell you: Nothing hits closer to home than when your mother has surgery in your own OR. As I gave out the cookies, everybody—the nurses, orderlies, patient floor clerks, housekeepers, anesthesiologists, and nurse anesthetists—were asking about my mother. It's not as though we're all close friends. We're colleagues. I said to one of the OR nurses, you're part of what made her surgery successful. I thanked the nurses on the floor for making my mother feel good. That was an important part of her experience.

No, it's not just the surgeon.

you have a private nurse, you may be off the other nurses' radar. They may figure that you're taken care of and therefore don't need them. Also, the private duty nurse may or may not have expertise in your particular problem. That's mostly the luck of the draw. To my knowledge, there's no list of nurse profiles from which you can simply select the best candidate.

Just as is true with other medical professionals, you are most assured of encountering a fine nursing staff by going to a fine medical institution. Less-than-stellar candidates will not be able to keep up with the pace and expectations. And, nurses who take pride in their work and want to perform at a high level will seek out the top places. In the larger, more sophisticated hospitals, nurses see the more complicated, interesting patients and therefore are always learning. This doesn't mean that other places have lesser quality nurses. In the better settings, you're almost always going to get a competent nurse.

The main rule in dealing with nurses is, don't be antagonistic. An irritable patient will get a response, to be sure, but it may not be exactly what he wants. Or he may get a response one time but not the next. Only be demanding when you need to be demanding. When it's an emergency, do whatever is necessary.

Also, to befriend your nurses, feed them! They're extremely busy and often don't get a chance to break for lunch. Give them something they can grab on the fly. It doesn't have to be homemade or fancy. Have something sent in your name to the nurse's station. Your gesture will be greatly appreciated.

When a friend of mine, whose mother was in the hospital, asked me how to get on the nurses' good side, I told her that food is a nice way to smooth the path. Her response was, "Great. I'll go out and buy a bunch of gourmet sandwiches." I said, "Forget it. The bread will be stale or soggy by the time they get a chance to sit down to them." Junk food is better, I told her. Donuts or something that comes in small pieces that they can nab as they rush by.

CHAPTER ELEVEN

The Patient's Advocate

W HEN YOU'RE WORRIED ABOUT YOUR HEALTH or the health of someone you love, you don't function effectively. When I'm wearing my physician's hat, I go on autopilot and can handle whatever comes my way. But when I was confronted with a medical emergency involving a close family member several years ago, I had to be jolted into gear.

I had just put my two young children to bed when the phone rang. A relative of mine was unable to rouse his wife from a nap. I rushed over and found her lying unconscious in bed.

As a physician, I had been in similar situations countless times. Had I been walking down the street in Manhattan and come across someone unconscious on the sidewalk, I would have immediately switched into professional mode and known exactly what to do. But this was a family member. I stood there, frozen. I didn't do CPR. I didn't call 911. I did nothing for what seemed an eternity, but was probably no more than one minute. Then I called her doctor, who told me to call 911. An ambulance arrived promptly and brought her to the hospital, where it was determined that the episode was brought on by a medication interaction. In the end, she was fine.

This was an unforeseen emergency, but the same holds true for other medical situations: your doctor finds a mass and wants to do a biopsy; your child has an accident. When it's personal, you can't think clearly. Even when you *think* you are thinking clearly, you're not. This is an important point to recognize. This is also why any time you're going to have surgery or face a difficult diagnosis, you need someone with a clear head to help you understand what's happening and make the best decisions. The issues we've discussed in this book—making sure you're seen by the appropriate doctor; weighing conflicting opinions; speaking up when you're not attended to—are extremely difficult to grapple with when you're under stress. You need someone to help you organize your treatment and your thinking. In short, you need an advocate.

WHAT IS AN ADVOCATE?

When I say advocate, I mean someone who can be by your side until the medical crisis or questions are resolved. This person will accompany you to visits to the doctor's office and to the hospital. He or she will listen to the doctor's prognosis and suggestions and take notes on key points. An advocate can also run interference for you, ensuring that your requests are fulfilled and dealing with the staff on scheduling matters, to relieve you of the added burden of logistics.

You certainly need an advocate when you're the patient. When there's something wrong with you, you don't hear everything that's said. First, it can be difficult to absorb information because you may be physically uncomfortable. And you may be somewhat shell-shocked from an emergency, diagnosis, or test result. I've found that, paradoxically, the more significant the information that the doctor is giving you, the more likely you are to zone out and miss it. Any time you're dealing with something more serious or more complex than an antibiotic for a straightforward infection, consider recruiting an advocate.

You also need an advocate when your child is seriously ill or needs surgery. As the parent, your job is to take care of your child—and yourself. You cannot expect yourself alone to reassure your child, calm your own nerves, *and* hear everything the doctor is saying. It's very difficult to listen to a doctor's comments when you're watching over your child and battling your own anxieties. If your child is hurting, you won't be able to get past your child's pain. This is not the time to be Supermom or Superdad. You need a second adult present to help you take in and process all the information.

CHOOSING YOUR ADVOCATE

The ideal candidate varies from person to person. Often a close relative—a brother, sister, son, daughter, father, or mother—is the best choice. But not always. Sometimes a spouse is your best option. However, it may be difficult for both of you to take time off from work. And the situation may be so emotionally fraught that your mate becomes counterproductive. When a child is the patient, the parents at times have a kind of emotional division of labor so that one parent nurtures the child and the other is able to distance himself enough to assume the role of advocate. You need to think about the psychological dynamics so that the advocate can truly be of help.

In every family, there's generally one person who understands medicine and how to navigate the system. These aren't always medical professionals per se. It's just that they intuitively sense how the field works and don't let the roadblocks stop them. They understand the politics of moving through a bureaucracy. This is the kind of know-how that makes for a good advocate.

Your advocate-to-be may be a personal or family friend. Perhaps someone you've known since you were schoolmates. Or someone at the office you just started getting to know a few months ago. You'll generally have a feel for who functions well in an emergency, who remains calm when everyone else is losing it, and who thrives on being helpful to others. You want someone who's reasonable, not someone prone to blow his stack. It's not always the obvious person. You might immediately think of your CEO master-of-the-universe friend who knows all the answers and is used to be in control. Wrong. Chances are that Mr. or Ms. CEO will assume they know more than they do, and may be reluctant to ask questions if they don't understand what the doctor says.

THE 'OTHER PATIENT'

It might seem natural for your spouse to be your advocate. I certainly wouldn't rule that out. But there are good reasons why it might be better to have another person assume this important role.

First, there's the simple emotional strain. If, God forbid, you become seriously ill, your mate is going to be riding the same emotional roller coaster as you. A serious illness has a huge emotional impact on a couple, more so than when one partner loses a job or nearly any other life event. For his or her own psychological self-preservation, a spouse may be tempted to downplay or deny problems. Or, his or her own concerns may begin to take center stage. Either way, it's neither productive nor helpful.

Choosing someone other than a spouse to be your advocate enables that person to perform an important, if unsung, role: to comfort and console your spouse. There is nothing more wretched than being alone in the hospital when your husband or wife is having surgery.

I think of the spouse or parents of a very sick patient as "the other patients." Usually, their needs fly beneath the radar. When I ask a patient's loved one, "How are you?" the response I often get is, "Nobody has asked me that before." I then tell them, "I want the real answer." And they say: "I'm terrible."

Someone needs to attend to the spouse of the patient. Everybody focuses on the patient—obviously. As well they sho uld. But the

You might think someone with sophisticated medical training would be the best. This is not necessarily so. I have a friend, Ronnie, who is not a doctor or nurse or therapist. She's a learning disabilities teacher, and she's one of those people who just *gets it*. When she's given complicated information, she generally understands it. When something doesn't sound right to her, she raises a question. No professional title or self-important manner intimidates her. She gets things done. The odds are that you know someone like this, someone sharp enough to catch what's being said, with the moxie to keep asking questions until he's satisfied.

---

wear and tear on the seemingly stalwart spouse—who's taking care of their mate, working to keep income coming in, caring for the children, and getting food on the table—is enormous. And according to our social conventions, they're not allowed to complain. They're supposed to smile bravely and never betray impatience with the often irritable patient who's in a lot of pain or extremely upset or even full of self-pity because something bad has happened to them. People forget that the bad thing happening to the patient is also happening to the spouse—and has transformed the spouse's role in the family.

I've noticed that if it's the wife who's sick, women in the community will offer the husband help with the kids and around the house. But in general, when the husband is sick, the wife doesn't get the same help—no doubt because she is expected to do all of that stuff anyway. Add a very sick spouse into the mix and no one, even a card-carrying Supermom, can function at 100 percent. It's very difficult. Wives often feel overwhelmed and alone, especially with long-term cancer patients. If someone is sick for a week, you can deal with it. You may be able to hide your feelings and do what you need to do. But when an illness drags on for months or years and you are forced to restructure your lives, the emotional impact is enormous.

Don't underestimate the toll this can take on you. Let the advocate assist you with the nuts and bolts of your medical care so that you can concentrate on your mate and yourself.

If, understandably, you are wary of asking an acquaintance or even a friend to take on the inconvenience of accompanying you to medical visits, consider this: You can offer to do the same for them. That makes it a fair trade.

First and foremost, you need your advocate to be someone who has your best interests at heart and doesn't have a personal agenda. That precludes "foul-weather friends" who gravitate toward those in misery because it makes them feel important. Or those who say, "How wonderful I am! Look how much I'm doing for you!" If you have an uncomfortable feeling about the arrangement, get out of it.

Sometimes the choice of who gets to be the point person for your care becomes competitive within the family—as with a patient with several adult children. Whoever isn't chosen may feel slighted. When someone falls ill, family pathology tends to kick up and create what a friend of mine aptly calls "genetic theater." People sometimes see tense medical situations as a chance to grandstand, or an opportunity to make up for past behavior. This is not the time. The decision about who advocates is neither about who loves you the most nor whom *you* love the most. It's strictly a matter of who can best represent your interests when you need an effective advocate, and who is available to provide this service.

It's important that one person is chosen. Advocacy by committee does not work in medical settings. People can get so caught up arguing about who is right that they forget about the patient.

If your choice of advocate angers your family or other friends or colleagues, tough. The person receiving the medical care, or the person responsible for a sick or injured child, gets to make this choice. No one else.

WHAT ADVOCATES DO

People often feel they should be able to handle medical matters on their own. They balk at the idea of finding an advocate, saying, "I don't want to bother anyone." Or they want to keep their problems private. Others hate the feeling of being in a vulnerable position, and don't like the notion of being the "sick" person in need of help from a "healthy" person. Drop any self-consciousness you may have about leaning on someone else. Choosing an advocate for your medical care is not a comment on your competence, intelligence, or inner strength. It is a practical response to the challenges of being a patient in a fast-moving, highly bureaucratized, extremely technical medical environment. It is a way of ensuring that you have backup when you need it and that all your needs and questions are addressed. It is simply being smart.

AN ADVOCATE PROVIDES YOU WITH COMPANY AND SUPPORT.

This person has to be able to take the time to go with you to doctors' visits, ongoing treatment, or the hospital during surgery. If someone else wants to come but can't, that's okay; it needn't reflect negatively on him or her. But your advocate must be absolutely reliable. Knowing that someone will be there for you alleviates your stress and also takes the pressure off other friends and family members who may not be so dependable.

Even when you're "fine," you should never have to sit alone in a hospital while waiting for a procedure. It's always nice to have someone with you, to see a familiar face when you're amidst a sea of unfamiliar faces. If you're waiting outside the operating room for your child, you need someone to be there for you. For any time a loved one is undergoing surgery, it's hard for you, too. When Len had his back surgery, I was on my home turf. I knew everyone involved in the surgery. The surgeon had my phone number in the pocket of his scrubs so that he wouldn't have to look for it. In essence, I stacked the deck as much as I could. But I knew that even that couldn't preclude the possibility that something could go wrong. I sat at my desk and tried to do paperwork. It was a waste of time. I was completely preoccupied. In these situations, you need someone to have a cup of coffee with. Or, someone to get a cup of coffee for you so that you aren't by chance gone at the moment the doctor comes.

Your advocate needs to have the temperament to deal with you either as the patient or as the parent of a very sick child, and to know what's right for you accordingly. This may mean offering solace should you get upsetting news. You can't have someone be a wimp about the whole thing. The advocate needs to be someone who's supportive and helpful and with whom you feel safe. You want to be able to let down your guard and express your fears. What you certainly *don't* want is to have to take care of the person who's allegedly taking care of *you*.

AN ADVOCATE HELPS YOU SECURE AND MANAGE INFORMATION RELEVANT TO YOUR MEDICAL CARE.

Patients (or the parents of patients) contending with a diagnosis or surgery have a lot of information thrown at them. Sometimes it comes so quickly that it's hard to take in fully. Many doctors go too fast. This is largely a matter of language. The doctor is speaking "medicine," itself a kind of shorthand. You're trying to hear everything *and* translate it all into English. Important: There's nothing wrong with saying to a doctor, "I don't understand, so will you please explain it a different way?" People think, "The doctor is so busy. There are twenty other patients waiting, so if I don't understand there must be something wrong with me." No, there's nothing wrong with you. It's your right to understand what your physician says to you, and the obligation of the physician is to explain it to you in terms you can understand.

Your advocate can play an invaluable role here. Trust me, no matter how sharp you are, if it concerns your health or your child's health you may not think straight or fast enough to know which questions to ask. Often you're left with a vague sense of confusion that hasn't quite been formulated as a question. Your advocate can take a read of your expression, see that you're not clear on things, and ask follow-up questions or urge the physician to reframe the issue at hand. Or you may think of a question the minute the doctor leaves.

If you and your advocate need things spelled out in a way that needs more time, you can ask if a nurse or someone in the office can answer some of the questions. Much of the material, such as postcare treatment, is fairly routine, and many doctors have assistants answer those kinds of questions. That's fine. What's more important is that the information comes to you in a form—and at a pace—that enables you to understand.

Many physician offices give you handouts about your diagnosis and treatment. These can be very helpful to ground you in the basics. Tell the office staffperson that you plan to go home and read the handouts, and ask (1) whom you can call later with questions; and (2) what time to call. Learn the information flow at that office. Doing things according to their terms will smooth your way.

Your advocate can help you process the information that you receive and then help you come up with appropriate follow-up questions. It's an axiom that you think of the best questions *after* the exam, like the witty retort you think of on your way home from a party. This is not a sign of failure on your part. You can regard your diagnosis and treatment as an ongoing conversation with your physician. Your advocate can help you refine your questions and encourage you to resolve them with your doctor.

Another reason an advocate is essential when you're gathering information is what I call "the Swiss cheese effect." By this I mean that each person's version of what the doctor says inevitably has holes in it. I remember some things and you remember other things. Ideally, the holes in your version are different from the holes in my version, so between us we can fill out the whole story!

The advocate can also handle all the nitty-gritty and take information down in the form of a medical diary. You can use a bound, loose-leaf book, index cards, or whatever system works for you. This is what goes in a medical diary: date; doctor seen; the doctor's contact information; why you're there; what is found; and the treatment recommended. I have one couple who wrote a diary entry of every one of their child's exams noting the vision treatments and my specific recommendations. This way they had a full dossier of my notes and during our conversations could refer back to examination results a year or two back.

One of the most important components of your medical diary is contact information. Be sure that your advocate records the

STRICTLY CONFIDENTIAL

Patient confidentiality is one of the bedrock principles of the medical profession. Your personal medical information is a matter between you and your doctor—and no one else. So if you want to bring an advocate along when you go in for treatment or consultation, you need to introduce him or her to your physician. Tell your doctor that this person is going to represent you, and that the doctor should talk to your advocate as if he were talking to you.

Be specific. Give the doctor your advocate's phone number and ask him or her to please call this person after your surgery. Also, make sure your doctors know that if they encounter your advocate in the hospital room, they should freely discuss your condition. If there is any question with regards to specific types of information, your doctor will speak to you. But if this is set up in advance, most doctors will not have a problem with it. More likely, they'll be grateful because there is someone responsible to whom they can pass along vital information.

names and contact numbers for every specialist that participates in your care. If you're in the hospital and a doctor comes in to take a look at you, you might think, "I'll remember who this person is." But it can start to build up. And in the twenty-four-hour world of the hospital, your sense of time can get blurred. You need to know each doctor's name, address, phone and fax number, as well as the date and time of the visit. You can simply take the physician's business card and jot down the time, and your advocate can record the visit in the log.

The basic data about the doctors you see are extremely useful. You may want to call the physician with questions. Or if you want to put your doctor in touch with one of the consultants, you can then provide not only the doctor's name but also a fax number. Your initial response may be, "It's not my job to act as secretary." Technically, that's true. But what you're doing is streamlining the record so that information gets across faster and with fewer chances for mix-ups. This is a small thing you can do to enhance your own care.

The documentation also becomes relevant for billing. One neighbor of mine owes his life to the doctors who cared for him after an emergency. Then the bills came. He had kept a record, so he could check with the doctors to determine that he had in fact been seen. One doctor said to him, "Oh, you're still here. I didn't even know that you had made it!"

Most doctors make hospital rounds very early in the morning. This does not mean that your advocate needs to report for duty by 7 A.M. You can arrange ahead of time for him or her to call and speak to a nurse in your doctor's office at a specified time to get the latest update. Just make sure that only one person calls in. You can't expect the office to report to your spouse, your mother, your friend, and so on. Keep the informational lines of command clean.

AN ADVOCATE HELPS YOU
NAVIGATE THE SYSTEM.

In medical settings, things go quickly—particularly in places like the emergency room. When you have to go to the ER, you may or may not have a friend or family member with you. It's best to have a designated advocate. But if not, the other person can assume that role.

When Margaret, my friend who had just had surgery, got sick, her husband brought her to the ER and the doctor took chest X-rays. As you may recall, nobody checked the X-rays and no one knew she had double pneumonia until several days later. Her advocate could have helped prevent this oversight by writing down all tests that were performed (for example, EKG, chest X-ray, blood tests), and then making sure that each test was accounted for before going home. An advocate would have asked, "What is the result of the X-ray?" or followed up with the pathology results. (X-rays can be read in a timely way; pathology results may take longer.)

When things are happening fast, you may forget that three things were done and one wasn't followed up. If it's written down, you can check each item. Margaret should have received better care several places along the way: (1) the covering surgeon should have helped out from the start; (2) she should have had an internist to follow her; and (3) the X-ray should have been read in the ER. She fell through the cracks. An advocate could have caught her before she fully slipped through.

A great deal of information comes out of the ER. You need to keep a list of tests that were done, doctors seen, and what the doctors found. And then another list of what you're expected to do: take medication, consult another doctor, take a diagnostic test. Make sure that the date and time you were admitted are written down, along with your patient identification number. This number is assigned to you as soon as you enter the hospital system, whether you're put in the ICU or taking a simple blood test. It will always be on all written documents pertaining to your care.

That number is yours forever. If you're in for a procedure, the number and your doctor's name will be on your wrist band.

AN ADVOCATE CAN HELP YOU GET WHAT YOU NEED.

As a patient, you may be reluctant to ask for what you need. That's where an advocate can come in.

There are strategies for getting whatever you may need in the hospital. Consider supplies such as towels, bed pads if you're bleeding, and extra plastic cups for drinking water. This is a low-level need. If the nurses aren't bringing something to you fast enough, you (or your advocate) can go to the nurse's station and politely ask for it. If nothing happens, you (or your advocate) can go and get it yourself. There's no dishonor in being a gofer. Should you be getting better service? Yes, but this is the real world.

If what you need is a narcotic to ease pain, as with Len after back surgery, then you need an advocate. Len politely asked for the narcotic—twice. Maybe the nurses were having an emergency down the hall and weren't able to respond. Maybe they had a list of priorities and simply didn't get to it. You can always go up the hierarchy, as I did. However, you need to pick your shots.

The hierarchy goes like this: There's the room nurse, an RN. The next level of authority is the head nurse on the floor, then the nursing supervisor. On top of all this is the hospital administrator on call. You or your advocate can obtain the phone numbers for all of these in an effort to represent a patient's interest. At the larger places, there is always someone onsite. At a smaller place, the administrator may not be in the hospital, but someone with a twenty-four-hour beeper is always in charge. If they can't address the problem, they have access to the person who can. We tend to regard going over someone's head as obnoxious. But when the patient's well-being is at stake, it is appropriate.

The first thing an advocate can do is set the stage for you to receive good care. It almost goes without saying, but this includes being polite to your caregivers. The last thing someone should do,

SET UP MEETINGS WITH YOUR DOCTOR

When a patient is in an intensive care unit, it's a good idea to set up a specific meeting time with the doctor. Doctors move in and out of the units quickly, and this way you know you'll see the doctor and won't feel like you're having a question hanging over you. Also, the doctor won't have to track you down when he or she wants to give you an update. It can be a timing disaster when the doctor goes looking for the family and they're down in the cafeteria or elsewhere.

There's a method to your doctor's seemingly random coming and goings, which may not be apparent to you. If you schedule a time to talk, it is easier for everyone. In between your meeting times, you can speak with the nurses, who are following the patient's minute to minute progress.

---

for instance, is brush aside an ICU nurse because you want your doctor. As we've seen, ICU personnel are high-level professionals who identify micro-changes in the patient's condition. They stay with the patient the entire time and know exactly what's going on.

Nurses work on a triage basis. The most attention is devoted to the patients who most need it. For example, right after Len's back surgery, the floor nurse was in the room almost the whole day. She was given fewer patients so as to make this possible. Sometimes you're on the wrong end of the triage system and you get less focused care. Your advocate will need to think clearly about the context. Are you really not getting what you need? Or are you simply not as sick as the guy in the next room? It helps to understand that the nursing staff is thinking according to the priorities of the floor unit as a whole. If you are not getting sufficient care to the detriment of your well-being, your advocate certainly has reason to intervene.

AN ADVOCATE KEEPS TRACK OF YOUR CARE.

If you're scheduled for an X-ray at 1 P.M. and nobody shows up, your advocate can check on what's happening. If you're supposed to have a certain medication for an IV drip, he or she can check that the right medication is being placed on the line.

This kind of follow-up can be extremely important. Once, my friend David's son was having back surgery and needed a blood transfusion. Before they gave the blood to his son, David—a fine ophthalmologist—double-checked and found that they had made a mistake: it was the wrong blood type. This was a potentially fatal error.

No matter how profoundly we wish it weren't so, mistakes will happen. Even in the finest hospitals, though in a major medical institution the odds are lower. What happened to David and his son sounds a clear warning for all of us: You should double-check any medication and blood that you receive. It is your right.

AN ADVOCATE CAN NOTICE PROBLEMS AND BRING THEM TO THE APPROPRIATE PERSON'S ATTENTION.

A friend of mine had a routine abdominal procedure in the morning. When she returned home in the afternoon, she was in extreme pain and asked her personal doctor friends for a narcotic. As pain is often telling of something amiss, we refused. She was quite sick with abdominal tenderness—and there shouldn't have been any. I stepped in as her advocate.

Her doctor was called, and she was told she was okay. But the pain progressed. On the third call to her doctor, after five hours had passed, I told the doctor that I was taking my friend to the emergency room—whether he made an appearance or not. (We also mentioned that my friend's litigator husband would be eager to meet him.) For one reason or another, her doctor met us in the ER.

It turns out that my friend had had a ruptured tubal pregnancy and had lost one third of her blood volume into her
abdomen. Ultimately, after she was operated on around 2 A.M.,
the bleeding was stopped, but it took her many months to recover
from the serious blood loss.

My friend was unable to call the doctor herself. Her pain and
discomfort overrode her ability to think clearly, so it was up to her
advocate to make the decision and take her to the hospital.

If this situation had been handled correctly by her physician,
she would have been seen again in her doctor's office in the late
afternoon and taken to the OR in the early evening. The delay of
seven hours to be seen and fourteen hours to have surgery resulted
in her extreme blood loss. Had she not been taken to the hospital
by her advocate, she would have gone into severe shock and quite
possibly died.

AN ADVOCATE CAN MAKE A FUSS WHEN YOU'RE EITHER UNWILLING OR UNABLE TO DO SO.

When Judy was giving birth, it was all she could do to manage the
contractions. Meanwhile, her husband, Tony, was keeping track
of everything else. He saw there was trouble with the fetal monitor, and while the labor and delivery nurse was initially resistant,
he firmly and politely insisted: "I'd like someone to look at this."
Once a different nurse took another look and saw that there was
a problem, an army of medical professionals descended on them.

Tony could have been mistaken. That's always a possibility
when an advocate makes a call. And a wrong call does hold a
risk: He could have antagonized someone whose help he needed.
Many people are mindful of that risk and are afraid to challenge
a professional or call attention to themselves or the patient for
whom they're advocating. But if you have a feeling—like Tony
did—act on it. You don't have to understand what's happening
or speak the language. If you're wrong, you're just the anxious
parent, friend, or patient, and there's nothing wrong with that.

And if you make the request politely and respectfully, you're unlikely to rub anyone the wrong way.

This is where I went wrong after hand surgery. I was reluctant to question my surgeon's judgment when he said that everything was fine. I knew that it wasn't fine. I should have mustered my courage sooner and said, "I want to be seen." Or had an advocate, who could have confirmed my doubts and urged me to make that step. Similarly, Julia's mother intuitively knew that her daughter's asthma was not improving under her current treatment. But she didn't know how to act on that knowledge. I had the distance to know that Julia needed to see someone else and stepped into the role of advocate to make that happen.

Do people ever overadvocate? Yes, family members can become belligerent. This is not helpful. This most commonly happens at the end of life. When the medical staff has determined there's nothing to be done, or the next of kin decides not to pursue aggressive treatment, someone often makes a stink. Legally, it is very clearly stated: The next of kin, the husband or wife or designated child, is the one to make the decisions. Everyone else's concerns are secondary. Often people who feel guilty toward the patient or are otherwise emotionally conflicted use this as a time to make amends. This is not the forum for that. When disagreements like this surface, the hospital staff looks like the bad guy. But the staff is honoring the most precious decision between the patient and the doctor. This is sacred. Nobody else gets to vote.

YOUR ADVOCATE: TRAFFIC COP AND PRESS SECRETARY

An odd thing frequently happens when someone becomes seriously ill: The patient becomes a host, and the illness an excuse for a party. That's why one of the advocate's jobs is to direct traffic around your hospital room and, during the post-op period, to deflect it from your home. Everyone comes to visit when what you really need is to be left alone to rest. This doesn't mean that there shouldn't be a few visitors. No one wants to be *that* alone. But it's difficult for the patient to say, "This isn't really a good time to see you." It's more comfortable when someone else can act as gatekeeper. The advocate can make it clear that the patient needs to rest, so visitors are allowed only at specified times. This eliminates potential sore feelings because everyone follows the same rules.

The same holds true if your child is ill or recovering from surgery. Your advocate needs to direct traffic so that you can attend to your child and not have to continually respond to well-wishers. You want to be able to read a book to your child, instead of running to answer a phone call from a well-meaning friend or relative. You don't have to take the calls. Nor does your spouse, who also needs to be free to concentrate on your child. Of course you appreciate others' concern, but answering the phone every time someone calls for an update eats up a lot of time and is exhausting, especially if you're already at your limit.

Which brings up another important job for an advocate, press secretary. You no doubt want to make sure that friends and relatives know how things are progressing; it's just that you don't want this to subsume all your energy. And it can. Your advocate can make and respond to calls for you. Important: How much information is shared is *your* decision, not someone else's, not your advocate's. Your advocate has to be willing to honor this, even if he or she knows more details than you're comfortable sharing.

A good way to manage this is via a telephone tree so that *your advocate* needn't be on the phone all day. In fact, there's nothing wrong with divvying up some of the responsibilities among other people to relieve your advocate of some of the burden. Just make sure that one person is coordinating things so that they all get done.

YOUR VOICE, YOUR HEALTH, YOUR LIFE

At the outset of this book, I discussed the importance of listening to your own voice when you feel some aspect of your care needs attention. Once you have an advocate, you have another voice to listen to—and another opinion to confirm your instincts when your own voice falters. When it comes to medical care, this is not a time to sit back. We all need to be informed, not only about our own condition but about how the system works. Many people regard this as a negative change. But throughout this book, we have repeatedly seen the benefits of a collaborative approach to medical care. Learning how doctors think is one part of this; understanding the importance of your decision-making is another. And assigning the role of advocate is yet another. These all help you take charge of your care in today's challenging medical environment.

APPENDICES

Medical Specialties: Member Boards and Associate Members

AMERICAN BOARD OF...

Allergy & Immunology
510 Walnut Street, Suite 1701
Philadelphia, PA 19106-3699
(215) 592-9466

Anesthesiology
4101 Lake Boone Trail, Suite 510
Raleigh, NC 27607-7506
(919) 881-2570

Colon & Rectal Surgery
20600 Eureka Road, Suite 600
Taylor, MI 48180
(734) 282-9400

Dermatology
Henry Ford Hospital
1 Ford Place
Detroit, MI 48202-3450
(313) 874-1088

Emergency Medicine
3000 Coolidge Road
East Lansing, MI 48823-6319
(517) 332-4800

Family Practice
2228 Young Drive
Lexington, KY 40505-4294
(859) 269-5626

Internal Medicine
510 Walnut Street, Suite 1700
Philadelphia, PA 19106-3699
(215) 446-3500

Medical Genetics
9650 Rockville Pike
Bethesda, MD 20814-3998
(301) 571-1885

Neurological Surgery
Smith Tower, Suite 2139
6550 Fannin Street
Houston, TX 77030-2701
(713) 441-6015

Nuclear Medicine
900 Veteran Avenue
Room 13-152
Los Angeles, CA 90024-1786
(310) 825-6787

Obstetrics & Gynecology
2915 Vine Street, Suite 300
Dallas, TX 75204
(214) 871-1619

Ophthalmology
111 Presidential Boulevard
Suite 241
Bala Cynwyd, PA 19004-1075
(610) 664-1175

Orthopaedic Surgery
400 Silver Cedar Court
Chapel Hill, NC 27514
(919) 929-7103

Otolaryngology
3050 Post Oak Boulevard
Suite 1700
Houston, TX 77056
(713) 850-0399

Pathology
P.O. Box 25915
Tampa, FL 33622-5915
(813) 286-2444

Pediatrics
111 Silver Cedar Court
Chapel Hill, NC 27514-1651
(919) 929-0461

Physical Medicine &
    Rehabilitation
3015 Allegro Park Lane, SW
Rochester, MN 55902-4139
(507) 282-1776

Plastic Surgery
Seven Penn Center, Suite 400
1635 Market Street
Philadelphia, PA 19103-2204
(215) 587-9322

Preventive Medicine
330 South Wells Street,
Suite 1018
Chicago, IL 60606-7106
(312) 939-2276

Psychiatry & Neurology
500 Lake Cook Road, Suite 335
Deerfield, IL 60015-5249
(847) 945-7900

Radiology
5441 East Williams Boulevard
Suite 200
Tucson, AZ 85711
(520) 790-2900

Surgery
1617 John F. Kennedy Boulevard
Suite 860
Philadelphia, PA 19103-1847
(215) 568-4000

Thoracic Surgery
One Rotary Center, Suite 803
Evanston, IL 60201
(847) 475-1520

Urology
2216 Ivy Road, Suite 210
Charlottesville, VA 22903
(434) 979-0059

ABMS ASSOCIATE MEMBERS

American Hospital Association
One North Franklin
Chicago, IL 60606-3421
(312) 422-3000

American Medical Association
515 N. State Street
Chicago, IL 60610
(312) 464-5000

Association of American
Medical Colleges
2450 N Street, NW
Washington, DC 20037-1127
(202) 828- 0400

Council of Medical Specialty
Societies
51 Sherwood Terrace, Suite M
Lake Bluff, IL 60044-2232
(847) 295-3456

Federation of State Medical
Boards
400 Fuller Wiser Road, Suite 300
Euless, TX 76039-3855
(817) 571-2949

National Board of Medical
Examiners
3750 Market Street
Philadelphia, PA 19104-3190
(215) 590-9500

Patient Bill of Rights

This notice is displayed prominently in my hospital and gives a good summary of the hospital's responsibilities and your own.

ALL PATIENTS HAVE THE RIGHT TO:

1. Understand and use these rights. If for any reason you do not understand or you need help, the hospital must provide assistance, including an interpreter.
2. Receive treatment without discrimination as to race, color, religion, sex, national origin, disability, sexual orientation, or source of payment.
3. Receive considerate and respectful care in a clean and safe environment free of unnecessary restraints.
4. Receive emergency care if you need it.
5. Be informed of the name and position of the doctor who will be in charge of your care in the hospital.
6. Know the names, positions, and functions of any hospital staff involved in your care and refuse their treatment, examination, or observation.
7. A no-smoking environment. Smoking is not permitted anywhere within the hospital.
8. Receive complete information about your diagnosis, treatment, and prognosis.
9. Receive all the information you need to give informed consent for any proposed procedure or treatment.

This information shall include the possible risks and benefits of the procedure or treatment.

10. Receive all the information you need to give informed consent for a Do-not-resuscitate order. You also have the right to designate an individual to give this consent for you if you are too ill to do so. If you would like additional information, please ask for a copy of the pamphlet "Deciding about CPR: Do-Not-Resuscitate Orders (DNR)," a Health Care Proxy form, or any Advance Directives.

11. Refuse treatment and be told what effect this may have on your health.

12. Refuse to take part in research. In deciding whether or not to participate, you have the right to a full explanation of the research program.

13. Privacy while in the hospital and confidentiality of all information and records regarding your care.

14. Participate in all decisions about your treatment in and discharge from the hospital. The hospital must provide you with a written discharge plan and written description of how you can appeal your discharge.

15. Review your medical record without charge and obtain a copy of your medical record, for which the hospital can charge a reasonable fee. You cannot be denied a copy solely because you cannot afford to pay.

16. Receive an itemized bill and explanation of all charges.

17. Complain without fear of reprisals about the care and services you are receiving and be provided with a written response. If you are not satisfied with the hospital's response, you can complain to the New York State Health Department. The hospital must provide you with the Health Department's telephone number.

A

B

C

E

local hospital versus major medical center, 29; nurses in, 186–187; pediatric, 36
emergency room nurses, 186–187
ER, 14, 147
examination, physical, what to do at, 58–62

F

floor nurses, 178–180
frozen sections, 167–170

G

Gawande, Atul, 130
general anesthesia, 136, 138, 140
generalist, second opinion from, 117–120
gifts for colleagues, 191
Gleason score, 92, 93, 166
Green, Ralph, 160–161

H

Harkness Eye Institute of Columbia, 144
Harvard Business School study, 129–130, 187
health care. *See* medical care
health information: finding, 43, 200–203; managing, 200–203
health insurance. *See* insurance
hematology, 162, 163
herbal preparations, telling doctor about all you are taking, 60
hierarchy: among doctors, 3, 10–13; medical, nurse's role in, 11; vertical, hospital's role in, 37

N

O

P

Q

R